OXFORD MEDICAL PUBLICATIONS

Burns

T0202094

Oxford Specialist Handbooks published and forthcoming

Oxford Specialist Handbooks in Surgery
Burns

Edited by

Iain S. Whitaker

Chair in Burns & Plastic Surgery, Swansea University
Medical School
Honorary Consultant Plastic Surgeon, The Welsh Centre
for Burns & Plastic Surgery
Deputy Editor, Journal of Plastic, Reconstructive and
Aesthetic Surgery (JPRAS)
Director, Reconstructive Surgery & Regenerative Medicine
Research Group (http://www.reconregen.com/)
SAC Lead, Academic Plastic Surgery

Kayvan Shokrollahi

Consultant Plastic Surgeon
Mersey Regional Burns and Plastic Surgery Unit,
Whiston Hospital, Liverpool, UK
Medical Director, The Katie Piper Foundation, UK
Editor-in-Chief: Scars, Burns & Healing Journal (SAGE)
Clinical Lead, Northern Burn Operational Delivery
Network, NHS England, UK

William A. Dickson

Consultant Plastic Surgeon and
Clinical Lead for the South West Burn Operational
Delivery Network (Adults), NHS England, UK

Editorial assistant
Nicholas Marsden
Registrar in Plastic Surgery Welsh Regional Centre for Burns and
Plastic Surgery, Morriston Hospital, Swansea, UK

OXFORD
UNIVERSITY PRESS

Great Clarendon Street, Oxford, OX2 6DP,
United Kingdom

Oxford University Press is a department of the University of Oxford.
It furthers the University's objective of excellence in research, scholarship,
and education by publishing worldwide. Oxford is a registered trade mark of
Oxford University Press in the UK and in certain other countries

First Edition published in 2019

Impression: 1

Published in the United States of America by Oxford University Press
198 Madison Avenue, New York, NY 10016, United States of America

British Library Cataloguing in Publication Data
Data available

Library of Congress Control Number: 2018966726

ISBN 978–0–19–969953–7

Printed and bound in China by
C&C Offset Printing Co., Ltd.

To my dearest Sara, my world, and to my parents without whose support I would never have made it this far.
KAYVAN SHOKROLLAHI

To my beautiful daughter Lara, who makes each and every day a joy, and my wife Sairan, who tolerates the countless hours of work.
IAIN S. WHITAKER

Foreword (UK)

'Sometimes wrong, never in doubt'

The often-quoted phase above concerning surgeons remains as true today as ever. *The Oxford Handbook of Burns* aims to reduce uncertainty and error by giving a contemporary, comprehensive and concise review of burn care.

Burn injury represents a global and systemic disease that requires a multidisciplinary approach to optimize survival, function, and aesthetic outcome. This is reflected in the multidisciplinary and multinational authorship of the book and acknowledges the vital contributions made to patient care by all members of the burn team. The Handbook reflects and incorporates the latest scientific knowledge, national guidelines, and international recommendations. Many of the authors are world authorities on their subjects and because of the book's format and size the reader does truly have an expert in their pocket.

In years to come it is the hope of the authors that the Handbook becomes a valued and trusted source for burn care professionals from whatever discipline to learn and update their knowledge and skills, prepare for exams, and to deliver excellent clinical care. For the more experienced practitioners, it is intended to be a useful and practical review that ensures up-to-date knowledge, particularly in areas outside areas of direct interest.

The book is aimed at all members of the burn multidisciplinary team to explain and inform on all aspects of care so that shared knowledge and understanding of treatment strategies and goals can improve collaboration and truly integrated care.

Peter Dziewulski
Consultant Plastic and Reconstructive Surgeon
St Andrews Centre for Plastic Surgery and Burns
Visiting Professor, School of Medicine, Anglia Ruskin University
Chelmsford, Essex, UK

Foreword (USA)

On Mondays and Thursdays, all the members of our practice make rounds together on all of our inpatients. We begin in the Burn Intensive Care Unit.

The plastic surgeons and nurse practitioners in our practice are joined by intensivists, a pharmacist, a member of our anesthesia team, our operating room team manager, a nutritionist, an infection control nurse, the hospital's chief nursing officer, our unit nurse manager, a case manager, physical and occupational therapists, our research director, respiratory therapists, and various students and visitors. Each patient is presented by the patient's nurse, and the discussion and planning draw input from the entire group.

It has often occurred to me during these rounds that I am practicing within the widest scope of care in my career. Ten years ago, more or less on a dare, I became the medical director of a private practice burn center in a state that had lost its only burn center some years previously and had been unable to organize burn care since. The president and chief surgeon of the Joseph M. Still Burn Center in Augusta, Georgia, invited me to organize a burn unit in Mississippi as an extension of his Georgia practice, which had been receiving burn patients from Mississippi while that state dithered in taking responsibility for the burn care of its own citizens.

The burn practice immediately engaged all functioning aspects of my training in general surgery and plastic surgery. I rapidly had to administratively organize clinics and inpatient units. Operatively, I proceeded to put together a network of nurse practitioners, clinic, hospital, and operating room staff as well as transfer protocols and consultants ranging from pediatricians to hospice care.

Personally, I had to upgrade my education base to a point where I could at least converse with the range of people involved in our burn practice. I had not practiced primary burn care since my plastic surgery residency (1984–1986). Drastic remedial instruction was necessary. Each month, I spent a week in the Augusta unit doing secondary burn reconstruction but, more importantly for me, observing and participating in burn care at that truly remarkable center which admits over 4,000 burn patients a year. Education was rapidly acquired.

Our Mississippi unit is now completing its tenth year, and I realize that this chapter of my career has made me a better physician and surgeon than perhaps I had intended. The acute and secondary care of people with burn injuries truly requires attention, responsiveness, a broad knowledge base, organizational skills, technical skills, and the ability to deal with the unexpected and unique problems that can be crucial to any burned patient.

This textbook embraces the great complexities of burn care and will be a valuable addition to my ongoing education. Scanning the table of contents, the reader will see the many elements of burn care arranged in a pattern equal to a complete profile of burn care. Systematic reading, or specific reading of particular topics, will give the reader the details of evaluation and management applicable to the complexities of burn care. The book will be immediately applicable to my practice.

As with all textbooks, this one will have missed evolving concepts and techniques by the time the book is published. The framework of this text, however, is a solid foundation for assimilating new information, so this first edition can be the beginning of many editions that may become a classic reference for burn care.

William C. Lineaweaver
Medical Director, JMS Burn and Reconstruction Center, USA,
Editor-in-Chief, Annals of Plastic Surgery, USA

Preface

Within these pages, we have concisely brought together the basic principles of holistic burn care for the generalist while at the same time catering for those working in specialist burns teams to provide a solid and accessible resource. We are especially pleased with unique features of the book such as the first publication known to us of a 'burn care formulary' of drugs used in the broad spectrum of indications relevant to burn patients, as well as various proformas and checklists helpful in day-to-day practice such as when referring or accepting burn patients.

Hence, the emergency physician will be reminded how to assess burn depth and body surface area accurately, and the plastic surgeon how to release and reconstruct burn scar contractures in a very substantial and well-illustrated chapter on this topic. The principles of rehabilitation and scar management receive substantial coverage also, as does specialist burns intensive care and anaesthesia.

Burns remain one of the commonest traumatic injuries, but thankfully the majority of these are relatively minor, a substantial proportion of which will be self-managed, managed in the community, managed in primary care, or managed in the emergency department. Burns experts should not lose sight of this skew. Similarly, even relatively small burns can result in serious and sometimes life-threatening or life-changing sequelae and require early specialist input, and this reminder is also worthy of note for generalists and front-line emergency services. We hope this textbook provides, among other things, a bridge between these two and a first port of call for all things burn-related.

Kayvan Shokrollahi, William A. Dickson,
and Iain S. Whitaker

Acknowledgements

We are most grateful to all our contributors who have helped bring this project to fruition.

OUP has been a truly professional publisher that has worked tirelessly to get the book over the line. Special thanks must go to Nick Marsden in his role as editorial assistant.

Finally, a personal word of thanks to all authors whose work we were, unfortunately, unable to include in the final manuscript.

Contents

Contributors

Ammar Allouni

Plastic Surgery Trainee, University Hospitals Birmingham NHS Foundation Trust, Birmingham, UK
Incidence and epidemiology, Cost of burn care

Francis Andrews

Consultant in Critical Care and Emergency Medicine, Whiston Hospital, Merseyside, UK
Critical care of burns patients

Ali Arham

Research Fellow, Shriners Hospital for Children, University of Texas Medical, USA
Chemical burns, Outcome measures for burns

Ernest Azzopardi

Senior Clinical Lecturer Swansea University Medical School, UK; Superspecialist Fellow in Laser Cutaneous Reconstruction, Laserplast SrL, Milan
Management of burn wound infection

Sarah Bache

Specialist Registrar in Plastic Surgery, St Andrew's Centre for Plastic Surgery and Burns, Chelmsford, Essex, UK
Burns surgery

Christopher Henry Barbara

Clinical Chairman, Pathology Department, Mater Dei Hospital, Malta
Management of burn wound infection

Greg Barton

Specialist Pharmacist Critical Care and Burns, St Helens and Knowsley Teaching Hospitals NHS Trust; Chair of the United Kingdom Clinical Pharmacy Association Critical Care Group (UKCPA CCG), UK
Burn care drug formulary

Kamal Bisarya

Resident, Burns and Plastic & Reconstructive Surgery, Imperial College Hospitals, London, UK
Military burns

David Bodansky

Plastic Surgery Trainee, Mersey Regional Centre for Burns and Plastic Surgery, Whiston Hospital, Liverpool, UK
Radiation burns

Peter Brooks

Consultant Plastic Surgeon, UK
Burns itch

Tania Cubison

Lieutenant Colonel and Consultant Burns and Plastic Surgeon, Queen Victoria Hospital, East Grinstead, UK
Military burns

Dallan Dargan

Plastic Surgery Trainee, Mersey Regional Centre for Burns and Plastic Surgery, Whiston Hospital, Liverpool, UK
Hand burns

Nagham Darhouse

Specialist Registrar in Plastic Surgery, Chelsea and Westminster Hospital, London, UK
Hair restoration

Baljit Dheansa

Consultant Burns and Plastic
Surgeon, McIndoe Burns Centre,
Queen Victoria Hospital, UK
*Outpatient management of minor
burns, Nutritional requirements in
the burn patients*

William Dickson

Consultant Plastic Surgeon and
Director of the Welsh Centre
for Burns and Plastic Surgery,
Morriston Hospital, Swansea,
Wales, UK
Remote assessment of burns

Peter Drew

Consultant Burn and Plastic
Surgeon, The Welsh Centre
for Burns and Plastic Surgery,
Morriston Hospital, Swansea, UK
Perineal and genital burns

Peter George Dziewulski

Consultant Plastic Surgeon,
St Andrews Centre for Plastic
Surgery and Burns, Mid Essex
NHS Trust, UK
*Burn depth assessment, Burns
surgery*

Shawn Fagan

Medical Director, Division of
Burns, Massachusetts General
Hospital, Boston, MA, USA
Hand burns

Celeste C. Finnerty

Associate Professor, Department
of Surgery, Sealy Center for
Molecular Medicine, University
of Texas, Texas, USA
*Hypermetabolic response to burns,
Chemical burns, Electrical injuries,
Outcome measures for burns*

Quentin Frew

Plastic Surgeon, St Andrew's
Centre for Plastic Surgery and
Burns, Chelmsford, UK
Burn depth assessment

Parneet Gill

Plastic Surgery Registrar, Countess
of Chester Hospital NHS
Foundation Trust, Chester, UK
Ocular burns

Nicole Glassey

Clinical Specialist
Physiotherapist, Burns and
Plastic Surgery, Nottingham
University Hospitals
NHS Foundation Trust,
Nottingham, UK
Occupational and physiotherapy

Jeremy Goverman

Division of Burns, Massachusetts
General Hospital; and
Assistant Professor of Surgery,
Harvard Medical School,
Boston, MA USA
Hand burns

Joseph Hardwicke

Associate Clinical Professor,
University of Warwick and
Consultant Plastic Surgeon,
University Hospitals of Coventry
and Warwickshire NHS Trust,
Coventry, UK
Burn wound dressings

Emily Hedges

Advanced Practitioner
Occupational Therapist,
Nottingham University Hospitals
NHS Foundation Trust,
Nottingham, UK
Occupational and physiotherapy

Sarah Hemington-Gorse

Consultant Burns and
Plastic Surgeon, The Welsh
Centre for Burns and Plastic
Surgery, Morriston Hospital,
Swansea, UK
*Predicting mortality and end of
life care, Sunburn and artificial
tanning*

David N. Herndon
Jesse H. Jones Distinguished Chair
in Burn Surgery, Professor of
Surgery and Pediatrics; Chief of
Staff and Director of Research,
Shriners Hospitals for Children,
Houston, TX, USA
*Hypermetabolic response to burns,
Chemical burns, Electrical injuries,
Outcome measures for burns*

Sandip Hindocha
Consultant Plastic Surgeon,
Clinical Director, Plastic
Surgery & Laser Centre.
Bedford Hospital NHS Trust
Desquamating skin disorders

Ranjeet Jeevan
Consultant Plastic Surgeon,
Manchester Centre for Plastic
Surgery and Burns, Manchester
University NHS Foundation
Trust, Manchester, UK
*The burns management pathway I,
The burns management pathway II,
Transfer proforma, Burn care re-
ferral criteria, Admission proforma*

Jong Lee
Associate Director of Burn
Services, University of Texas
Medical Branch, Houston,
TX, USA
Electrical injuries, Paediatric burns

Jorge Leon-Villapalos
Consultant in Plastic Surgery and
Burns, Lead Clinician, Chelsea
and Westminster Hospital;
Senior Honorary Clinical
Lecturer, Imperial School of
Medicine
Burns first aid

Karen J. Lindsay
Plastic Surgery Registrar,
Aberdeen Royal Infirmary,
Aberdeen, UK
Tetanus, Laser management of scars

Nigel Tapiwa Mabvuure
Plastic Surgery Registrar, East of
England Deanery, Broomfield
hospital, Chelmsford, UK
*Pathophysiological response to
burns, Chemical burns, Outcome
measures for burns, Outpatient
management of burns, Nutritional
requirements in the burn patients*

Nick Marsden
Specialist Registrar, the Welsh
Centre for Burns and Plastic
Surgery, Morriston Hospital,
Swansea, UK
*Predicting mortality and end of life
care, Sunburn and artificial tanning*

Walter J. Meyer III
Professor, Department of
Psychiatry and Behavioural Sciences,
University of Texas Medical Branch,
Galveston, TX, USA
Pain management

Anuj Mishra
Consultant Plastic Surgeon,
Manchester Centre for Plastic
Surgery and Burns, Manchester
University NHS Foundation
Trust, Manchester, UK
*The burns management pathway II,
Burn care referral criteria,
Admission proforma*

Naiem Moiemen
Consultant Plastic Surgeon
and Director of the Healing
Foundation UK Burns Research
Centre, Birmingham, UK
*Incidence and epidemiology, Burn
wound dressings, Cost of burn care*

Adeyinka Molajo
Specialty Registrar in Plastic
Surgery, Department of Burns
and Plastic Surgery, St Helen's and
Knowsley NHS Trust, Whiston
Hospital, Merseyside, UK
*Non-accidental injury (NAI) in
children*

Christopher F. Munson
Clinical Research Fellow,
Canniesburn Plastic Surgery
Unit, Glasgow Royal Infirmary,
Glasgow, UK
*Pathophysiological response to
burns, Nutritional requirements in
the burn patients*

William B. Norbury
Reconstructive Burns Fellow,
Shriners Hospital for Children,
University of Texas Medical
Branch, USA
Escharotomies

Michael Peck
Associate Director, Arizona
Burns Centre, Phoenix, AZ, USA
Burn prevention

Jonathon Pleat
Consultant Burns and Plastic
Surgeon, North Bristol NHS
Trust, Bristol, UK
*Pathophysiological response to
burns*

Bohdan Pomahac
Associate Professor of Surgery,
Harvard Medical School, Boston,
MA, USA
Face transplantation

Sophie Pope-Jones
Specialist Registrar, The Welsh
Centre for Burns and Plastic
Surgery, Morriston Hospital,
Swansea, UK
Remote assessment of burns

Tom S. Potokar
Chair in Global Burn Injury &
Director NIHR Global Health
Research Group on Burn
Trauma, University of Swansea,
UK; Honorary Consultant Plastic
Surgeon, Welsh Centre for
Burns & Plastic Surgery, UK
Principles of burn reconstruction

Rowan Pritchard-Jones
Consultant Plastic Surgeon,
St Helen's & Knowsley
Teaching Hospitals NHS Trust,
Liverpool, UK
*Assessment of burn surface area,
Fluid resuscitation in burns,
Remote assessment of burns*

Rene Przkora
Associate Professor of
Anesthesiology and Pain Medicine
Department of Anesthesiology
College of Medicine, University
of Florida, Gainesville, FL, USA
*Hypermetabolic response to burns,
Pain management*

Alison Reeves
Senior Physiotherapist, Burns
and Plastic Surgery, Nottingham
University Hospitals NHS
Foundation Trust, Nottingham, UK
Occupational and physiotherapy

Norbert Schrage
Department of Ophthalmology,
County Hospital Cologne,
Cologne, Germany
Ocular burns

Chris Seaton
Research Manager, Virtual
Machine Group, Oracle Labs, UK
Fluid resuscitation in burns

Kayvan Shokrollahi
Consultant Burns and Plastic
Surgeon, Mersey Burns
Centre, Whiston Hospital,
Merseyside, UK
*The burns management pathway I,
The burns management pathway II,
Assessment of burn surface area,
Fluid resuscitation in burns, Skin
substitutes, Burns scar management,
Non-accidental injury (NAI) in chil-
dren, Desquamating skin disorders,
Frostbite, Laser management of
scars, Transfer proforma, Burn care
referral criteria, Admission proforma*

Indranil Sinha
Fellow in Burn Surgery, Division
of Plastic Surgery, Brigham and
Women's Hospital, Harvard
Medical School, Boston,
MA, USA
Face transplantation

Sujatha Tadiparthi
Consultant Plastic and
Reconstructive Surgeon,
Queen Elizabeth Hospital,
Birmingham, UK
Skin Substitutes, Frostbite

Raj M. Vyas
Plastic Surgeon, Division of Plastic
Surgery, Brigham and Women's
Hospital, Harvard Medical School,
Boston, MA, USA
Face transplantation

James Warbrick-Smith
Registrar, The Welsh
Centre for Burns and Plastic
Surgery, Morriston Hospital,
Swansea, UK
*Perineal and genital burns,
Principles of burn reconstruction*

Stuart B. Watson
Consultant Plastic
Surgeon, Canniesburn Unit,
Glasgow Royal Infirmary,
Glasgow, UK
Burn contracture surgery

Greg Williams
Hair Transplant Surgeon, Farjo
Hair Institute, London, UK
Hair restoration

Lee C. Woodson
Chief of Anaesthesiology,
Shriners Hospital for Children,
University of Texas Medical
Branch, Galveston, TX, USA
*Anaesthesia: preoperative
management of patients with
acute burns, Anaesthesia:
intraoperative management of
patients with acute burn injury,
Pain management*

William L. Yancey
Department of Anaesthesiology,
University of Texas Medical
Branch, Galveston, TX, USA
Pain management

Susie Yao
Plastic Surgery Registrar,
Specialist Registrar,
Mersey Burns Centre, Whiston
Hospital, Merseyside, UK
*The burns management pathway I,
The burns management
pathway II, Transfer proforma,
Admission proforma*

Christina Yip
Canniesburn Plastic Surgery
Unit, Glasgow Royal Infirmary,
Glasgow, UK
*Outpatient management of minor
burns*

Chapter 1

Incidence and epidemiology

Introduction to incidence and epidemiology

Burns are a global public health problem. The World Health Organization (WHO) estimated that 11 million people worldwide required medical care in 2004.[1] Approximately 300,000 people die each year from fire-related burns (not including deaths from scalds, electrical injuries, chemical, and other types of burns). The majority, over 95% of these burns, occur in low- and medium-income countries (LMICs). Fire-related mortality is 11.6 deaths per 100,000 population per year in South East Asia, 6.4 in the Eastern Mediterranean, and 6.1 in Africa, compared with approximately one death per 100,000 population per year in the developed countries.[2]

In the UK an average of 13,000 people each year are admitted to hospital with burn injuries, while in the USA 410,000 burn injuries occurred in 2008, with approximately 40,000 requiring hospitalization.[3] The peak age incidence (Fig. 1.1) is between 20 and 50 years. In India over 1 million people are moderately or severely burned each year, while in Bangladesh, Colombia, Pakistan, and Egypt, 18% of children with burns have a permanent disability. Causes of burns are tabulated in Table 1.1 showing that the incidence of flame burns in LMICs is almost double that in developed countries.

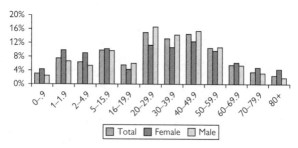

Fig. 1.1 Age category distribution of 163,771 patients in 91 hospitals in the USA from 2001 to 2010. Y-axis is the percentage of the total burns.

Table 1.1 Burn aetiology

Type of burn	USA[1]	UK[2]	Australia[3]	India[4]
Flame burn	42%	37%	37%	77%
Scald burn	34%	28%	33%	14%
Contact burn	9%	19%	7%	–
Electrical burn	4%	11%	5%	7%
Chemical burn	3%	3%	18%	2%

Source: Data from (1) ABA National Burn Repository. Report on data from 2005 to 2014, Copyright © American Burn Association 2014, available from http://www.ameriburn.org/NBR. php; (2) International Burn Injury Database. UK Burns Injury Data 1986–2007 Inc., UK National Burn Care Group, Copyright © IBID 2008, available from http://www.ibidb.org/downloads/cat_view/913-ibid-reports; (3) Greenwood JE, et al. Increasing numbers of admissions to the adult burns service at the Royal Adelaide Hospital 2001–2004. ANZ Journal of Surgery 77(5):358–63, Copyright © 2007 Royal Australasian College of Surgeons; and (4) Ahuja RB, et al. Changing trends of an endemic trauma. Burns 35(5):650–6, Copyright © 2009 Elsevier Ltd and ISBI. Published by Elsevier Inc. All rights reserved.

Risk groups

Children

Over half of burned children are under the age of 5 years and almost a third are under the age of 2 years. In the under 1 year olds, scald burns are the most common thermal injury, followed by contact burns, with flame being very uncommon. However, flame burns are the commonest type of burns in children 10 years or older (Fig. 1.2).

Elderly (>65 Years)

Elderly burned patients represented an average of 14% of hospital admissions in the USA from 1991 to 2005, data published from the US National Burn Repository. As life expectancy in many of the developed countries is over 80 years (78.2 in USA and 80.1 in UK), there is an increased incidence of burns in elderly people, with female predominance over the age of 75 years. Flame burns in this age group are the most common, followed by scalds. Burns mostly happened in the bedroom or the bathroom. The

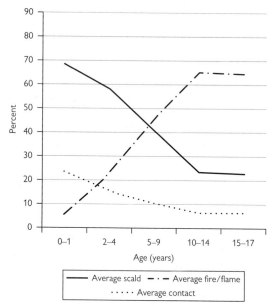

Fig. 1.2 Incidence of burns in children.

Reproduced from Kramer CB, et al. Variations in U.S. pediatric burn injury hospitalizations using the national burn repository data. Journal of Burn Care Research 31(5):734–9, Copyright © 2010 The American Burn Association, with permission from Oxford University Press.

average length of stay is 2.8 days/% total body surface area (TBSA) for the 65–75 age group and 3.3 for the older patients. Half of patients aged 65–75 were discharged home while only one-third of patients older than 75 were discharged home. Likewise, 16% of 65–75 year olds died in hospital and 24% of older patients died in hospital.

The disabled

Underlying physical or cognitive disabilities because of medical conditions such as epilepsy, peripheral neuropathy, cardiac dysrhythmia, or TIA (transient ischaemic attack) can lead to burns, especially in the elderly population. In addition, the presence of pre-existing comorbidity affects patients' outcomes and mortality (Table 1.2).

The disadvantaged 'socioeconomic factors'

In a study of a national cohort of 870,411 of burned patients in North Korea, burn injury severity was significantly affected by the socio-economic status. Lack of family support especially in children has been shown to affect post injury life re-adjustments.

Patients with psychiatric disorders, alcohol, substance abuse, or smoking

Psychiatric history and substance abuse has a two-way cause–effect relationship with burns. Two-thirds of all burn patients have at least one psychiatric disorder. These patients have a longer length of stay and poor adjustment following acute care. Smoking and substance abuse also increase the risk of sustaining a burn more than six times the normal population. There is also evidence of delayed wound healing as a result of stress.

Table 1.2 Relationship between comorbidity, age, and outcome

Characteristic	No. of comorbidities			
	0	1	2	3+
Percentage of patients	73.6	15.0	7.1	4.3
Age (years) (mean)	40.4	47.9	54.5	60.3
Length of stay (days) (mean)	11.5	15.9	17.8	21.7
Died in hospital (%)	5.4	8.8	13.0	19.4

All differences among groups defined by number of comorbidities are significant (P < 0.001).

Non-accidental burns

Non-accidental injuries include neglect and intentional injuries. This can affect children and vulnerable adults. In children, parental drug abuse, single parent families, delay to presentation, and lack of first aid were statistically more prevalent in burns due to neglect. These burns are statistically more likely to be deeper and require skin grafting. Intentional burns in children vary between 1% and 3% of all paediatric burns admissions. Burns due to child neglect were reported to be up to 8% of hospital admissions.[4] The care of almost half of these children was transferred to foster parents.

Mass casualties

Burn disasters during the twentieth and twenty-first centuries, excluding terrorist attacks, have shown a trend of reduced fatalities per disaster as a result of strict preventative legislation. Historically, in most fire disasters, victims die immediately with fewer than 50 casualties with severe burns requiring hospitalization. Table 1.3 shows the distribution of burns victims in selected terrorist attacks.

Table 1.3 Selected terrorist attacks

Year	Incident	Location	Injured	Burns	Fatalities
1982	Coal Mine Explosion,	Cardowan	40	36	0
1982	Hyde Park Bombing,	London	23	5	3
1983	Harrods Bombing,	London	91	7	6
1984	Coal Mine Explosion,	Abbeystead	44	44	16
1984	Refinery Explosion,	Pembrokeshire	16	16	4
1984	Oxford Circus Station Fire,	London	15	15	0
1984	Putney Gas Explosion,	London	10	10	8
1985	Ship Explosion, Milford Haven,	Wales	13	13	3
1985	Stadium Fire,	Bradford City	253	250	53
1985	Plane Crash,	Manchester	137	2	52
1985	M6 Coach Crash,	Lancashire	27	2	13
1987	Kings Cross Fire,	London	45	24	29
1988	Piper Alpha Explosion,	North Sea	25+	25+	165
1989	Car Bombing,	Peterborough	>100	2	1
1992	Castleford Chemical Plant,	Yorkshire	18	3	2
1993	Littlewoods Store Fire,	Chesterfield	30	30	2
1994	Smithfield Cinema Fire,	London	12	12	11
1998	Bombing,	Omagh	336	7	29
1999	Soho Nail Bombing,	London	81	Several	3
1999	Paddington/Ladbroke Grove Train Crash,	London	447	>30	31
2001	Steel Plant Explosion,	Port Talbot	15	Several	3
2005	Buncefield Fuel Depot Fire,	London	43	43	0
2006	July 7 Bombings,	London	700	40	54
2009	Lakanal Tower Fire,	London	20+	20+	6
2015	Shoreham Air Crash,	West Sussex,	13	13	11
2017	Grenfell Tower Fire,	London	64*	2*	72*

*est

Further reading

Park JO, Shin SD, Kim J, Song KJ, Peck MD. Association between socioeconomic status and burn injury severity. Burns 2009;35:482–90.

Pham TM, Kramer CB, Wang J, Rivara FP, Heimbach DM, Gibran NS, Klein MB. Epidemiology and outcomes of older adults with burn injury: an analysis of the National Burn Repository. Journal of Burn Care and Research 2009;30:30–6.

References

1. WHO. Burns. Key facts. http://www.who.int/mediacentre/factsheets/fs365/en/. Accessed 21 September 2015.
2. WHO. Injury chartbook: a graphical overview of the burden of injuries. http://www.who.int/violence_injury_prevention/publications/other_injury/chartb/en. Accessed 25 September 2015.
3. British Burn Association. National burn care review 2001. http://www.britishburnassociation.org/nbcr. Accessed 25 September 2015.
4. Chester DL, Jose RM, Aldlyami E, King H, Moiemen NS. Non-accidental burns in children—are we neglecting neglect? Burns 2006;32:222–8.

Burn prevention

Definition of burns

A burn is an injury to the skin or other organic tissue primarily caused by thermal or other acute trauma. It occurs when some or all of the cells in the skin or other tissues are destroyed by hot liquids (scalds), hot solids (contact burns), or flames (flame burns). Injuries to the skin or other organic tissues due to radiation, radioactivity, electricity, friction, or contact with chemicals are also identified as burns.

Haddon matrix categorizes risk factors

Burn injuries result from an interaction of the human host, the agent of energy transfer, and the physical and social environment in which the event occurs. Use of the Haddon matrix[1] describes the factors responsible for burns in terms of the time sequence of events (Table 2.1).

- Factors in the pre-event phase can be avoided using primary prevention techniques that prevent the burn from occurring
- Factors in the event phase can be ameliorated using secondary prevention techniques that minimize the damage caused by the energy transfer
- Factors in the post-event phase can be amended using tertiary prevention techniques that improve survival, functional, and cosmetic outcomes from the burn injury

Table 2.1 Haddon matrix applied to risk factors for residential fire burns and death

Factors→ Phases↓	Host (person)	Agent	Physical environment	Socioeconomic environment
Pre-event	Smoking in bed Chronic alcoholism Debilitated elderly	Flammable substances stored in house Young children with access to matches or lighters	Frayed electrical wiring Overcrowding Absence of functional smoke alarms	Lack of or poorly enforced building codes Poverty, unemployment, illiteracy
Event	Lack of escape plan Inappropriate response to alarms	Absence of sprinkler systems or fire extinguishers Absence of fire retardants in clothing and household materials	Bars on windows No ladder for upper story rooms	Insufficient legislation or enforcement for smoke alarm or sprinkler installation Inadequate community infrastructure for requesting emergency services
Post event	Ignorance of appropriate first aid		Shortage of emergency medical transportation	Inadequate access to burn centres for treatment and rehabilitation Paucity of community support for recovery

Categories of burn prevention countermeasures

These strategies represent the ways in which the transfer of energy can be controlled, modified, or interrupted:
- Prevent the creation of the hazard
  - Ban manufacture and sale of unsafe products
  - Prohibit unsafe practices
- Reduce the amount of energy in the hazard
- Prevent the release of a hazard that already exists
- Modify the rate or spatial distribution of the hazard
- Separate the hazard from those to be protected, in space or time
- Separate the hazard by a material barrier
- Modify relevant basic qualities of the hazard
- Make what is to be protected more resistant to damage from the hazard
- Counter the damage done by the hazard
- Stabilize, repair, and rehabilitate the one damaged by the hazard

Third dimension of Haddon matrix

Decision-making for selection of burn prevention intervention strategies can be facilitated by the use of value criteria:
- Effectiveness
- Cost
- Freedom
- Equity
- Stigmatization
- Preferences
- Feasibility

In general, implementation of burn prevention programmes takes place through the three Es:
- Enforcement of legislation or regulations
- Education
- Engineering and design modification

Monitoring and evaluation

Ongoing appraisal of the process and outcomes is critical to the success of any burn prevention programme.

- Understanding of scope and magnitude of burn problem
  - Epidemiological pattern
  - Major causes
  - Risk factors
- Documentation of effectiveness of programmes
  - Cost–benefit ratio
  - Modification vs. discontinuation of unsuccessful programmes
- Future directions
  - Continuation and expansion of successful programmes
  - Resource allocation

Examples of successful strategies

Several burn prevention programs have documented effectiveness, including epidemiological studies, controlled trials, and evidence of sustained decreases in population-based burn rates.[2]

Child-resistant lighters

- Nature of the problem—many residential fires (and associated burns and deaths) are caused by children playing with cigarette lighters and matches
- Solution—ignition mechanism can be designed to prevent operation by children under 5 years of age
  - For example, depression of the metal shield is required before the flywheel can be turned to make a spark
- Implementation of the solution—U.S. Consumer Product Safety Commission developed standards in 1994
  - Nearly 60% reduction in childhood injuries and deaths caused by playing with lighters in the USA following implementation
  - Similar standards in UK, EU, Canada, Australia, and New Zealand[2]

Electrical safety

- Nature of the problem—increasing electrification of low- and middle-income countries is associated with concurrent upsurge in electrical injuries and structure fires
- Solution—both engineering design and regulations play a role in prevention of electrical injury, including
  - Insulation of wires
  - Fuse and circuit-breaker systems
  - Safe routing of electrical wires within and between structures
- Implementation of the solution
  - Underwrites laboratory tests and standardizes safety features of electrical products, and National Fire Protection Agency publishes and updates National Electrical Code
    - —Ground fault circuit interrupter shuts off electrical device when escape of current is detected, preventing electrocution
    - —Arc fault circuit interrupter disconnects device when arc is detected, preventing fires
    - —Occupational Safety and Health Administration mandates workplace safety standards
    - —Employee training in electrical theory
    - —Safe work procedures
    - —Hazard identification
    - —Proper use of protective equipment
    - —First aid and rescue techniques[2]

Child nightware safety

- Nature of the problem—clothing can be ignited by contact with stoves, heaters, cigarettes, or other sources of flames; very serious burns occur when children's sleepwear ignites

- Solution—fabrics can be made less flammable by increasing the content of synthetic material, by making clothes tight-fitting, and by adding flame-retardant chemicals
- Implementation of the solution—The nightware (safety) regulations 1985 was amended to minimize the risk of ignition of children's sleepwear and reduce the speed at which fire would spread after ignition occurred
  - The National Fire Protection Agency estimates that there was a 10-fold reduction in children's sleepwear deaths after implementation of the standards[2]

Fire-safe cigarettes

- Nature of the problem—cigarettes are frequent ignition sources for structure fires
  - Each year in the USA there are over 700 deaths from fires caused by cigarettes
  - In the European Union in 2006, cigarettes caused 650 deaths and €48 million in property damage
- Solution—cigarettes can be manufactured so that they self-extinguish when not being smoked, and thus are less likely to ignited clothing, bedding or furniture if dropped
- Implementation of the solution—legislation has been passed in the USA, Canada, Australia, European Union, South Africa, and many countries of the former USSR
  - Attempts at Federal legislation in the USA failed in the 1970s because of opposition from the tobacco industry
  - Eventual success in the USA was due to passage of State laws, beginning in 2004 in New York
    - Smoking material fire deaths in New York State decreased by 40% after implementation of the law[2]

Fireworks safety

- Nature of the problem—pre-adolescent and adolescent boys are at greatest risk, sustaining not only burns, but blast injuries to the hands and eyes
- Solution—local or state legislation bans or restricts the sales of fireworks
- Implementation of the solution
  - Regulation of fireworks sales in the UK and Denmark—particularly when combined with education programmes—has reduced the number of fireworks injuries
  - Repeal of legislation in Minnesota led to resurgence of injuries[2]

Regulation of hot water heaters

- Nature of the problem—scald burns caused by hot water are among the most common types of burns, particularly in very young children
- Solution—reducing the temperature of water, the duration of exposure, or both will diminish the depth of burn and severity of injury
- Implementation of the solution—setting the temperature regulators of hot water heaters to keep hot tap water below 120°F (50°C) has been shown to reduce the number and severity of paediatric scald burns[2]

Smoke alarms

- Nature of the problem—housefires account for majority of burn deaths in high-income countries (HICs)
- Solution—early detection of heat, smoke or carbon monoxide gives occupants time to escape
- Implementation of the solution—education campaigns and enforcement of legislation has led to implementation of installation and maintenance of smoke alarms[2]

Sprinklers

- Nature of the problem—structure fires in the USA caused over 2,700 deaths and resulted in $9.7 billion in direct property damage in 2010
- Solution—sprinkler systems detect fire and douses it with water, limiting its spread
  - Risk of death from residential fire is 80% lower in homes with sprinklers
  - Property damage in structures protected by sprinklers is 1/5 the damage in unprotected structures
- Implementation of the solution—legislation and enforcement of regulations are necessary to bring about widespread installation of residential sprinkler systems
  - Homeowners and the construction industry are resistant to additional costs
    — Sprinkler installation increases the cost of a new home by $1–2 per square foot
    — Retrofitting a home costs about the same amount as laying new carpet
  - Only 2% of family homes in the USA are protected by sprinklers[2]

References

1. Haddon W. The changing approach to the epidemiology, prevention, and amelioration of trauma: the transition to approaches etiologically rather than descriptively based. American Journal of Public Health 1968;58:1431–8.
2. World Health Organization. Burn prevention: success stories and lessons learned. Geneva: WHO; 2011.

Pathophysiological response to burns

Understanding the pathophysiological response to burns

An understanding of the pathophysiological responses to burns has underpinned advances in care and outcomes. Burns result in local and systemic changes which affect organs distal to the focus of injury.

Local responses to burns

The model proposed by Jackson considers the local response to burns in three concentric zones (see Fig. 3.1). The 'zone of coagulation' is where irreversible necrosis of skin has occurred. Surrounding this there is the 'zone of stasis' where the tissue has sustained a sub-critical insult. Anti-inflammatory agents and vasodilators may prevent progression to necrosis in this area. Wound healing begins from the outermost 'hyperaemic zone'. Vessels in this area are dilated to facilitate the delivery of immune components including cells and mediators such as cytokines.

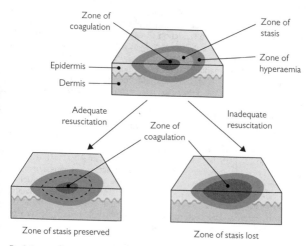

Fig 3.1 Jackson's burn zone model.

Reproduced with permission from Hettiaratchy S, Dziewulski P. ABC of burns: pathophysiology and types of burns. The British Medical Journal 328(7453):1427–9, Copyright © 2004, British Medical Journal Publishing Group.

Systemic changes

Multisystem changes occur following large burns (>20–30% TBSA).

Cardiovascular function and burn shock

Burn shock occurs when organ function is compromised by reduced perfusion. The mechanisms leading to burn shock are a complex interplay between hypovolaemia and several inflammatory mediators released post-burn, such as histamine (see Table 3.1).

Heat disturbs vascular endothelial and cell membrane integrity. Increased microvascular permeability allows leakage of fluid from the intravascular space, which becomes hypovolaemic, to the interstitial space, where it causes oedema. Insensible fluid losses are also increased secondary to evaporation following loss of epithelial barrier function. Homeostatic compensation is attempted by a rise in peripheral vascular resistance. These changes contribute to the reduction of cardiac output (CO) immediately post burn. However, CO falls before hypovolaemia occurs, suggesting a simultaneous direct neurogenic response. Further, the myocardium may be depressed by a mediator released by burn wounds, although this is not yet fully characterised. Cardiac dysfunction in the first two days (ebb phase) further stimulates release of inflammatory mediators – a positive feedback cycle.

The kidneys receive 25% of cardiac output and are therefore sensitive to reductions in circulating volume. Hypovolaemia leads to pre-renal acute kidney injury and, potentially, renal failure which can have a mortality rate of 88% for adults and 56% for children.

Early and adequate fluid resuscitation is crucial in ameliorating the effects of burn shock. However, since inflammatory mediators including a myocardial depressant factor contribute to burn shock, correcting hypovolaemia alone does not entirely obviate the problem. Further, although patients with extensive burn require large amounts of fluid, resuscitation should be closely monitored since restoration of circulating volume can exacerbate oedema caused by hyperpermeable vessels.

Effect on metabolism and inflammation

A stereotyped neuroendocrine response occurs following trauma. This response is possibly an evolutionary adaptation to mobilise energy sources, primarily glucose for the 'fight or flight' response. Neural excitability results in increased secretion of catabolic hormones such as cortisol and glucagon, anti-insulin hormones such as growth hormone (GH) and catecholamines. In concert, these hormones cause hyperglycaemia by inducing glycogenolysis and gluconeogenesis. Gluconeogenic substrates are derived from lipolysis and proteolysis partially explaining lean muscle loss and cachexia. This stress response to trauma is clinically indicated by tachycardia, pyrexia and elevation of serum neutrophil and inflammatory markers, e.g. CRP (C-reactive-protein).

A systemic immunoendocrine response also occurs following large burns and other critical illnesses. Transcriptome analysis shows that similar genes are activated secondary to endotoxaemia, blunt trauma, and burns. However, the response to burns is massively amplified and proportionate to burn size. Post-burn immunoendocrine changes persist beyond wound

Table 3.1 Mediators of burn injury

Mediator	Role
Histamine	Released from mast cells and increases early phase microvascular permeability by inducing gap formation between endothelial cells
	Increases capillary pressure and fluid extravasation by dilating arterioles and constricting venules
Prostaglandins	Derivatives of arachidonic acid released from burned tissue and inflammatory cells such as activated macrophages and neutrophils
	Vasodilatory and increase microvascular permeability
Thromboxane	Produced locally by platelets
	Can cause progression of partial-thickness to full-thickness injury through vasoconstriction
Kinins	Local inflammatory mediator that contributes to fluid shifts by increasing venular permeability
Serotonin	Released early following burn injury
	Contributes to the rise in peripheral systemic resistance by constricting the smooth muscle of large vessels
Catecholamines	Adrenaline and noradrenaline released is augmented following burn injuries
	These catecholamines reduce capillary pressure by constricting arterioles. They may also limit histamine- and bradykinin-induced capillary permeability. These two actions encourage fluid reabsorption from the interstitium
	Potentiate hypermetabolism and hyperdynamism of the circulation
Oxygen radicals	Activated neutrophils release oxygen free radicals including the superoxide anion, hydrogen peroxide and hydroxyl ion
	These contribute to fluid shifts by damaging microvascular endothelial cells and thus increase vascular permeability
Platelet aggregation factor	Contributes to oedema by increasing capillary permeability
Angiotensin II and vasopressin	Regulators of fluid balance and potent vasoconstrictors of terminal arterioles
	Increased release following burns
	Angiotensin II implicated in selective gut mucosal ischemia with subsequent translocation of bacteria and endotoxins, sepsis, and potential multi-organ failure
	Vasopressin, with catecholamines, is likely largely responsible for increased system vascular resistance which increases left heart afterload and, therefore, cardiac work

Data sourced from Jeschke M. Pathophysiology of burn injury, p. 13–29, in Jeschke MG et al. (eds) Burn care and treatment. Vienna, Austria: Springer. Copyright © 2013; and Keck M, et al. Pathophysiology of burns. *Wiener Medizinische Wochenschrift* 159(13–14):327–36. Copyright © 2009 Springer-Verlag Wien.

closure for up to 3 years. These changes are associated with adverse outcomes such immune incompetence and associated sepsis, increased fracture risk, growth retardation, reduced organ function, impaired wound healing, and death.

The primary mediators of the hypermetabolic response are catecholamines, glucocorticoids, and inflammatory cytokines, such as the pro- inflammatory interleukins (IL) 1 and 6. These mediators remain elevated for up to 36 months post burn. Jeschke et al. compared several hypermetabolic and inflammatory parameters in 977 burned children (>30% TBSA) and 107 age-matched controls. Predicted resting energy expenditure (REE) was significantly greater in burned children from injury up to 2 years post burn, indicating prolonged hypermetabolism. Up to 2000-fold rises in proinflammatory cytokines (IL 6 and 8) and chemokines (granulocyte-colony stimulating factor (CSF) and monocyte chemoattractant protein-1) were recorded for 36 months. Levels of catecholamines, glucocorticoids, acute-phase proteins, and other cytokine were also elevated to varying extents and lengths of time (see Table 3.2).

Serum hormone panels are also deranged following large burns. For example, growth hormone, parathormone, oestradiol, and testosterone levels may be reduced whereas progesterone levels are elevated. Insulin levels are significantly elevated but sustained hyperglycaemia suggests an insulin-resistant state. Elevated levels of catabolic hormones such as catecholamines, cortisol, and glucagon, as well as increased glycolysis and gluconeogenesis, also cause hyperglycaemia which is linked to immune dysfunction and increased risk of infections.

Table 3.2 Summary of hypermetabolic and inflammatory derangements following large burns (>30% TBSA)

		Magnitude of difference	Duration (months)
Catecholamines	Urinary adrenaline	5-fold	18
	Urinary noradrenaline	10-fold	2
Glucocorticoids	Serum and urinary cortisol	Up to 10 fold	36
Cytokines	G-CSF, MCP-1, IL-6, IL-8	Up to 2000 fold	36
	IL-1β, -2, -5, -7, -10 and -17, TNF-α, IFN-γ, GM-CSF	up to 20-fold	Most of the 36 month study period
Acute-phase proteins	CRP	13-fold	9

G-CSF, granulocyte-colony stimulating factor; MCP-1, monocyte chemoattractant protein-1; TNF-α, tumour-necrosis factor-alpha; IFN-γ, interferon-gamma; GM-CSF, granulocyte-macrophage; CRP, C-reactive protein; IL-interleukin.

Data sourced from Jeschke MG, et al. Long-term persistence of the pathophysiologic response to severe burn injury. Plos One 2011;6(7):e21245. Copyright © 2011 Jeschke et al. This is an open-access article distributed under the terms of the Creative Commons Attribution License, which permits unrestricted use, distribution, and reproduction in any medium, provided the original author and source are credited.

Table 3.3 Effects of losses of lean body mass (LBM)

Magnitude of LBM loss (%)	Effects
10	Immune dysfunction
20	Decreased wound healing
30	Increased risk for pneumonia and pressure sores
40	Possible death

Body composition and organ changes secondary to hypermetabolism
The hypermetabolic and hyperinflammatory stress response produces long-term changes in body composition and organ function.

Bone mineral content, lean body mass, fat content, height, and weight were all significantly reduced in burned children for 36 months post burn.

Loss of lean body mass results from muscle protein catabolism which is increased to provide gluconeogenic substrates. However, since the sequelae of low LBM can be fatal (see Table 3.3), pharmacological and nutritional interventions are important to ameliorate proteolysis. A similarly multifaceted approach including anabolic agents—such as oxandrolone and growth hormone (GH)—and physical therapies is required to correct post-burn osteopenia.

In burnt children, the liver remains almost double the size of controls with correspondingly elevated transaminases, alkaline phosphatase, and reduced albumin. Hepatomegaly is associated with increased septic susceptibility and mortality risks.

Effect on other systems

Burns can also adversely affect other systems directly or indirectly (see Table 3.4).

Gastrointestinal mucosal atrophy occurs early and affects absorption of glucose, fatty acids, and amino acids. Intestinal permeability is also increased, increasing the risk of sepsis. Furthermore, intestinal blood flow decreases. These changes, along with post-burn ileus, reduce the body's capacity to absorb nutrients required to support the hypermetabolic states. Early enteral feeding is crucial to ameliorate these changes in an effort to avoid potentially catastrophic malnutrition.

The immune system is also globally depressed following burns. The scale of immune depression is proportional to burn size. Burn patients, by virtue of lost skin barrier function, are susceptible to microbial colonization. Immune incompetence further reduces the capacity to mount responses. Patients become susceptible to a range of infective complications which can be fatal. Sepsis remains the largest cause of post-burn mortality.

Pulmonary function is also adversely affected by burn-induced oedema, regardless of whether inhalation injury is present. Burns increase pulmonary vascular resistance and wedge pressures. This, combined with neutrophil and TNF-α-mediated increases in pulmonary microvascular permeability, encourages fluid shifts. Both hypoprotenaemia, from plasma protein loss through the burn wound, and overzealous fluid resuscitation also increase risk of pulmonary oedema. Reduced airway compliance and impaired gaseous exchange occurs. Respiratory function could also be affected by proteolysis of intercostal and accessory muscles of respiration secondary to hypermetabolism.

Table 3.4 Summary of the effects of burn injury on key systems

Cardiovascular	
Early phase	*Hypermetabolic phase*
Hypoperfusion	Hyperperfusion
↑ Capillary permeability	Oedema
↑ Peripheral vascular resistance	Cardiac arrhythmias
↓ Cardiac output	Mycocardial dysfunction
Renal	
Early phase	*Hypermetabolic phase*
Hypoperfusion	Hyperperfusion
↓Glomerular filtration rate	↑Glomerular filtration rate
	Acute renal failure
Respiratory	Gastrointestinal
Pulmonary hypertension	Paralytic ileus
↑ Airway resistance	Gastric stasis
↓ Compliance	GI ulceration
	GI haemorrhage
	↓ Mesenteric perfusion
	↓ Nutritional absorption
	Bacterial translocation
	Hepatic hypoperfusion

Further reading

Jeschke M. Pathophysiology of burn injury. In Jeschke MG, Kamolz L-P, Shahrokhi S (eds) *Burn care and treatment*. Vienna: Springer, 2013; pp. 13–29.

Jeschke MG, Gauglitz GG, Kulp GA, et al. Long-term persistence of the pathophysiologic response to severe burn injury. Plos One 2011;18;6.

Jeschke MG, Mlcak RP, Finnerty CC, et al. Burn size determines the inflammatory and hypermetabolic response. Critical Care 2007;11:R90.

Keck M, Herndon DH, Kamolz LP, et al. Pathophysiology of burns. Wiener Medizinische Wochenschrift 2009;159:327–36.

Hypermetabolic response to burns

Hypermetabolic response to burns

Although improvements in clinical care have been made over the past three decades and these improvements have translated into reduced morbidity and mortality, a large thermal injury remains one of the most disastrous injuries today.

The burn survivor experiences not only several psychosocial stressors and disfigurement, but also a unique metabolic response to the trauma that does not resolve with burn wound closure and healing. This problem has been best studied in paediatric burn patients.

These hypermetabolic and catabolic responses are seen in patients with burns over more than 30% of the total body surface area (TBSA). Two phases are observed:

- The 'ebb' phase starts immediately after a burn, lasts 2–3 days, and is characterized by a 'shock state' with decreases in cardiac output, oxygen consumption, metabolism, and glucose tolerance
- The 'flow' phase starts approximately 5 days after a burn. This phase can last up to 3 years (the maximum follow-up period reported) in paediatric patients with >30% TBSA burned. The flow phase is characterized by persistent hypermetabolic and inflammatory responses, leading to catabolism and loss of function, which delay re-integration of the burn survivor into society

Findings:

- Metabolism: Indirect calorimetry is used to quantitate hypermetabolism. The resting metabolic rate increases immediately post burn to 180% of the basal rate during the acute phase, is 110% at 12 months, and remains elevated up to 3 years post burn. Heightened glycogenolysis, gluconeogenesis, and lipolysis create an environment of elevated glucogenic precursors, resulting in hyperglycaemia and insulin resistance. Hyperglycaemia itself is associated with a higher infection rate, which in turn exacerbates metabolism and catabolism. Serum triglycerides and glucose levels increase gradually during the flow phase and remain elevated even after wound healing is complete. These elevations, which can also last for up to 3 years, are associated with peripheral lipolysis and insulin resistance
- Body composition: Catabolism (characterized by muscle wasting, a negative nitrogen balance, weight loss, and decreased bone mineral content) can be so severe that growth arrest can result. Metabolic studies have shown that muscle protein is broken down to fuel the hypermetabolic response. Without intervention, a lethal loss of 20–25 mg/m^2 nitrogen can be reached in 2–3 weeks after a severe burn
- Organs: Cardiac output increases after the ebb phase. Studies in paediatric patients with >30% TBSA burns have shown that cardiac output remains increased for up to 12 months after a burn before returning to age-matched, non-burned, normal values. An increase in liver size, as measured by ultrasound, occurs in paediatric burn patients and does not return to normal even after 3 years

- Inflammatory response: Many cytokines and acute-phase proteins are elevated after a burn. Dramatic changes have been observed for IL-6, IL-8, G-CSF, and MCP-1, with increases of up to 2,000-fold compared to non-burned control levels. GM-CSF, INF-γ, TNF-α, IL-1β, IL-2, IL-5, IL-7, IL-10, and IL-17 increase significantly above control levels and have been found to remain elevated for most of the 3-year follow-up period. Alterations in serum acute-phase proteins include elevations of serum complement C3, haptoglobin, α1-acidglycoprotein, and CRP, with decreases in α2-macroglobulin. Expression of serum constitutive hepatic proteins such as transferrin, retinol-binding protein, and pre-albumin are lower in burn patients than in controls. Hepatic enzymes are elevated with concurrent decreases in albumin
- Hormonal imbalance: Urinary catecholamines and cortisol are elevated immediately after a burn and remained elevated. Norepinephrine is elevated up to 540 days post burn. Decreases in growth hormone, insulin growth factor-1, insulin-like growth factor binding protein-3, and parathyroid hormone occur as well

Additionally, infections and sepsis are associated with significant increases in metabolism and oxygen consumption, which may underlie adverse outcomes after a burn.

Strategies to attenuate hypermetabolism and catabolism

Improvements in the acute care regimen, such as aggressive fluid resuscitation, have dramatically decreased burn mortality over the last two decades. In addition, these interventions attenuate the hypermetabolic and catabolic responses.

- Early excision and grafting: In patients with large burns (>50% TBSA), excision and grafting within 2–3 days of the trauma reduce the metabolic rate by 40% compared to the rate in burn patients not undergoing wound coverage until 1 week after injury. Catabolism is greatly reduced in these patients as well. In patients undergoing complete excision and wound coverage within 72 hours of injury, the net protein loss has been reported to be 0.03 μmol of phenylalanine per minute per 100 mL of leg blood volume compared to 0.07 μmol in patients who undergo excision 10–21 days after a burn. Cadaver skin or biosynthetic skin substitutes are equally effective for immediate burn wound coverage

- Nutrition: A better understanding of the nutritional requirements of burn patients has improved outcomes and reduced the incidence of the once-common post-burn sequelae of significant weight loss. Early enteral feeding initiated within 1 day of the injury attenuates the metabolic–catabolic response. Interestingly, intravenous feeding or delayed enteral feeding after the acute phase does not provide this beneficial effect. The intravenous route should be reserved for scenarios in which enteral feeding is not possible such as ileus. Nutritional requirements are increased after a burn and can be established using a metabolic cart to prevent over- or underfeeding. Importantly, the post-burn metabolic–catabolic response is prolonged, thus the nutritional requirements should be measured at regular intervals to ensure continued optimal nutrition

- Environmental warming: Loss of insulating skin and reset of the body temperature to 2°C above normal after a severe burn further enhances hypermetabolism and catabolism. Simply increasing the environmental temperature (room temperature) to 28–33°C decreases resting energy expenditure from 2.0 to 1.4 in patients with >40% TBSA burns, thus decreasing hypermetabolism

- Treatment of infection: Prompt treatment of infections and sepsis decreases catabolism, morbidity, and mortality. Septic burn patients have a 40% increase in metabolic rate and catabolism compared to non-septic patients with a similar burn size

- Pain and anxiety: Burn patients experience prolonged and constant pain related to their injury. This pain is initially nociceptive in nature but increasingly neuropathic components evolve during the healing process. Additionally, burn patients undergo frequent painful procedures such as dressing changes, debridement, intravenous line placements, and physical therapy, all of which cause a significant increase in pain. Adequate and prompt pain control and treatment of anxiety decrease the stress response and the associated negative metabolic effects

- Pharmacological modulation of the response: Investigational drug therapies have been shown to successfully attenuate the hypermetabolic and catabolic responses to a burn. Recombinant human growth hormone (rHGH) increases protein synthesis, muscle mass, weight, height, and bone mineral content, while decreasing wound and donor site healing time. Recombinant HGH increases serum concentrations of insulin-like growth factor 1 (IGF-1) and insulin-like growth factor binding protein 3 (IGFBP-3), which mediate the effects of rHGH. Administration of IGF-1 together with IGFBP-3 produces similar effects
- Androgenic hormones such as testosterone and oxandrolone have been used to attenuate the post-burn hypermetabolic and catabolic responses. Oxandrolone appears favourable as it has only 10% of the masculinizing potency of testosterone. Additionally, oxandrolone can be given via the enteral route, whereas rHGH is administered intramuscularly or subcutaneously. Oxandrolone is also more cost-effective than rHGH. Oxandrolone improves height (in paediatric burn patients), weight, lean mass, and bone mineral content. Insulin therapy to maintain euglycaemia during the post-burn acute phase decreases hyperglycaemia, improves protein synthesis and muscle mass, and attenuates the proinflammatory response. Insulin also improves wound healing. Concerns regarding hypoglycaemia during insulin administration have led to the investigation of other hyperglycaemia-attenuating approaches including metformin, fenofibrate, and glucagon-like peptide 1 (GLP-1). The efficacy of these drugs is currently being studied in on-going trials. As systemic catecholamines are elevated for several years after a burn injury, studies of β-adrenergic receptor blockade with propranolol have demonstrated improvements in body composition with increased net protein synthesis, increased muscle mass, and a decreased inflammatory response. The administration of propranolol for a full year is now being investigated
- Combination therapies using drugs with complementary action, such as oxandrolone with propranolol or growth hormone with propranolol, have been studied in small groups of patients with positive effects and can also be considered
- Exercise: A physical therapy program is essential to rehabilitate a burn patient by replacing the lost muscle and restoring function. Exercise is necessary to increase protein synthesis and uptake into the muscle. Resistance exercise programs produce better outcomes, such as increased lean mass, strength, and function, than standard rehabilitation programs. Exercise also enhances the positive effects of the previously mentioned anabolic pharmacological approaches

Summary

Hypermetabolism and catabolism are typical responses to a severe burn injury and can persist for several years. Early interventions including excision and grafting of wounds, enteral feeding, treatment of infections, and pharmacological interventions (eg. anabolic hormones, adrenergic receptor antagonists) and exercise can successfully attenuate this otherwise deleterious response.

Further reading

Jeschke MG. Postburn hypermetabolism: past, present, and future. Journal of Burn Care Research 2016;37:86–96.
Diaz EC, Herndon DN, Porter C, et al. Effects of pharmacological interventions on muscle protein synthesis and breakdown in recovery from burns. Burns 2015;41:649–57.

The burns management pathway I: assessing and transferring patients with an acute burn injury

The acute burn injury

Burns lead to critical injuries that may, if inadequately or inappropriately managed, result in multiple organ dysfunction and death.

Early management is undertaken almost exclusively by individuals with relatively little experience in assessing and treating burns. In this chapter we highlight the important steps in initially managing and safely transferring burns patients to a specialist burns unit.

Initial management at scene

Initial management involves:
- Safely extricating the patient
- Administering appropriate first aid measures
- Analgesia
- Urgent transfer to the nearest emergency department

Burned areas should be:
- Exposed and cooled with copious amounts of cold water
- Wrapped with a protective dressing (eg. cling film)
- Covered along with the rest of the patient to maintain the patient's body temperature during transfer

For chemical burns:
- Avoid direct contact
- Brush off any excess if a dry chemical
- Administer specific antidotes immediately if available
- If an antidote is not available, lavage with copious amounts of water for a prolonged period; steps should be taken to ensure that this will not cause an adverse reaction

For electrical burns:
- First aid should not be commenced until the patient is extricated to a place of safety

---

Note

First aid cooling with water is temporary and stops on withdrawal from the water source. Cooling with cold packs is widely used but acts beyond the therapeutic window can subsequently reduce the patient's core temperature contributing to hypothermia. Cold packs should be applied for a maximum time of 30 minutes.

Transfer to the local emergency department

Paramedic ambulance crews should immediately transfer patients to the nearest emergency department (ED) or trauma centre, and should not attempt direct transfer to a distant specialist burns unit.

The paramedic team should:
• Take a history from the patient and any witnesses
• Protect the airway and cervical spine
• Administer high flow oxygen where indicated
• Provide appropriate analgesia
• Keep the patient warm
• Obtain an electrocardiogram and initiate cardiac monitoring for patients with an electrical burn
• Inform the receiving emergency department of the incoming transfer

All standard basic and advanced life support assessment and treatment measures should be taken, in particular those outlined by the Advanced Trauma Life Support (ATLS®) and Emergency Management of Severe Burns (EMSB) protocols.

Management of major burns at the local emergency department

Initial management should include:
- ABC's and exclusion of other non-burn injuries
- Anaesthetic assessment of the airway
- Early intubation if indicated
- Cervical spine protection
- Administration of high flow oxygen unless contraindicated
- Application of an oxygen saturation measurement probe
- Arterial blood gas measurement, including carbon monoxide levels
- Wide bore peripheral venous access, through unburned skin where possible
- Fluid resuscitation (see below)
- Cardiac monitoring
- Sending venous blood for standard investigations
- Measurement or estimation of the patient's weight
- Early placement of an urinary catheter
- Regular assessment and management of pain
- Monitoring and maintaining the patient's core and peripheral temperature
- Drying the patient and removing any cooling agents.
- Minimizing exposure to that required to undertake a full secondary survey
- Assessing the depth and extent of the burns
- Elevating limbs with circumferential burns and considering the need for escharotomies; these are ideally performed at a specialist burns unit if transfer times are minimal, but seek advice and undertake them emergently in life or limb threatening scenarios
- Appropriate dressings
- Considering placement of a nasogastric tube
- Administering human tetanus toxoid and/or immunoglobulin
- Other investigations as indicated

Arrangements should be made for urgent transfer to the nearest specialist burns unit/centre with an available intensive therapy or ward bed as required. In the UK, the National Burns Bed Bureau will assist in finding a bed, and similar coordinating bodies are present in many other countries.

Special considerations

In patients at risk of abuse or non-accidental injury, the local emergency department should raise any concerns and initiate appropriate local referral pathways. This should not delay the patient's transfer to a specialist burns unit for definitive management.

Assessment of burn area and depth at the local emergency department

The priorities for the ED physician are to:
• Rapidly assess and manage the burned patient
• Ensure no other specialist involvement is required due to co-existent injury
• Identify the receiving specialist burns unit
• Communicate details of the patient and their injuries to them
• Transfer them safely after instituting all essential early interventions
• Do so in a way that minimizes the risk of hypothermia

The size and depth of the burn should be estimated to guide initial fluid resuscitation. This should be done once and effectively to avoid unnecessary exposure of the patient and hypothermia. The assessment of burns depth is discussed in more detail later in this Handbook (see Chapter 10).

Erythematous skin without blistering should be excluded from all fluid calculations, with the caveat that burns can deepen with time and significantly alter injury severity. Skin with partial thickness burns is usually soft, blistered, painful, may be moist, and blanches on direct palpation or pressure. Skin with full thickness burns is usually painless, stiff, white, brown or black in colour, dry and leathery, and may be charred with eschar.

The areas of the patient's body with partial or full thickness burns should be accurately recorded on a Lund and Browder chart (Appendix 1) and the overall percentage should then be estimated (see Chapter 9).

Circumferential burns to the neck, torso and limbs should be identified and documented as they may require early escharotomies.

Initiating fluid resuscitation at the local emergency department

The patient should be resuscitated using the modified Parkland formula if the burn involves more than 15% of the total body surface area (TBSA) in adults and 10% in children.

Fluid should be given as Hartmann's or Ringer's lactate. In children, maintenance fluid should also be administered as dextrose/saline. If the patient presents late, fluid due in the hours following the burn injury but prior to presentation may be given as a single bolus if not contraindicated, or over the remainder of the first 8-hour resuscitation period (this can be discussed with the accepting burns unit).

Fluid resuscitation over first 8 hours post injury
  (For adults >15% TBSA burn, Children >10% TBSA burn only)
  0.25 mL × % TBSA burn × weight (kg) = mL/hour
  (Hartmann's solution)
  This is based on 3–4 mL/% TBSA burn/kg in the 24 hours **post injury** (not presentation), with half given over the first 8 hours. A catch-up bolus may be required (please check with accepting unit).
  The free Mersey Burns App will assist clinicians in estimating the % TBSA and calculating fluid requirements (www.merseyburns.com).

Paediatric cases: In addition to fluid resuscitation, paediatric patients also require maintenance fluids using a dextrose/saline solution (such as 5% dextrose and 0.45% sodium chloride):
4 mL/kg for the first 10 kg plus ...
2 mL/kg for the second 10 kg plus ...
1 mL/kg for each additional kg
This is the volume of maintenance fluid required hourly (in mL/hour) in the 24 hours post injury.

Burns injuries should not prevent or delay the emergency department from resuscitating the patient as per the ATLS® protocol when they first arrive. The volume of any fluid bolus given on arrival should simply be deducted when calculating the initial hourly fluid prescription using the modified Parkland formula.

Referring patients to a specialist burns unit

All patients with burns injuries may be discussed with a specialist burns team. In the UK, the National Network for Burn Care has produced guidelines for the referral of burns to specialized burn care services, which are provided in Appendix 2.

Essential referral information to ensure safe patient transfer

Once the decision has been made to transfer the patient, this should be undertaken promptly and safely to minimize the risk of the patient deteriorating en route to the burns unit, on what may be a long distance or cross-regional transfer.

The referring member of staff should ensure that:

- The transfer proforma is completed
- Any pre-transfer assessments and treatments requested by the specialist burns team have been undertaken
- The patient is reassessed systematically to confirm that their airway remains patent and that their physiological status has not changed since initial presentation
- Appropriate fluid resuscitation has been initiated and will continue during the transfer
- Initial first aid adjuncts applied to cool the patient (such as cold packs) have been removed after the first 30 minutes to prevent hypothermia
- The transferring ambulance crew has the appropriate equipment and expertise, with an accompanying medical escort if indicated.
- Copies of all medical notes, drugs and fluid charts, investigation results and imaging are sent with the patient
- Priority is given to arranging a speedy transfer to a burns service with an available bed, while maintaining the patient's body temperature

The burns management pathway II: receiving and initially managing a patient with burns

The burns multidisciplinary team

Medical

One or more specialist burns surgeons should lead the multidisciplinary team that cares for burns patients. Junior medical staff will be actively involved in care delivery and training.

Nursing

Experienced specialist burns nurses should lead a team of dedicated nursing and ancillary staff responsible for ward-based patient monitoring and care, as well as outreach in some circumstances.

Intensive care and anaesthesia

One or more specialist burns anaesthetic and critical care doctors should be an integral part of the team. Their role includes initial airway assessment and management following transfer, providing supportive care to help prevent and treat single or multiple organ dysfunction and sepsis, and pain management. Specialist anaesthetic management during burns surgery is vital as it presents unique challenges.

Operating theatre

Burns surgery should be undertaken in a dedicated operating theatre with a specialist surgical, nursing, and ancillary team that regularly dresses, excises, and grafts acute burns injuries, performs associated procedures such as tracheostomy, and undertakes secondary burns reconstruction. Specialist equipment including that required to warm the patient (overhead heaters, climate controlled heating) is a prerequisite of a burns operating theatre.

Rehabilitation

Specialist rehabilitation is essential following a burns injury to minimize recovery time and optimize the functional outcomes attained. Burns physiotherapists work collaboratively with medical and nursing staff to ensure active and passive mobilization and early and optimal functional recovery. Occupational therapists undertake numerous activities including splinting, pressure garment provision, and discharge planning. Play specialists may also help to rehabilitate children.

Clinical psychology

Specialist clinical psychologists are important in helping to assess and counsel burns patients for both pre-existing psychological conditions and de novo problems related to their injury, its aetiology and its sequelae. Liaison with psychiatric services is often required.

Dieticians

Nutritional support is critically important in the burn population, many of whom require supplemental feeds. These are usually provided through gastric or jejunal feeding tubes but occasionally via a parenteral route.

Receiving and accepting an acute burn referral

Burns referrals are generally taken via telephone by the burns unit medical and/or nursing staff. As the experience of these staff members may vary, it is helpful to use a standardized proforma to collect information about the patient, their burns and any associated injuries, the treatments provided and their planned transfer (Appendix 1). Written criteria for accepting a referral should also be available to these members of staff (Appendix 2).

Essential referral information to collect and record

- Patient name and date of birth
- Contact details of referring unit and individual
- Time of referral
- Date and time of burns injury plus fluid administered so far
- Mechanism of burns injury (including any inhalational component, associated injuries or acute medical issues)
- First aid administered at time of injury
- Estimated burn percentage (of total body surface area)
- Patient weight in kilograms
- Assessments and investigations completed and current physiological status (eg. results of primary and secondary survey, bloods, ECG, radiographs, scans)
- Treatments initiated and completed (eg. intubation, supplemental oxygen, intravenous access and fluid administration, analgesia, human tetanus immunoglobulin, burns irrigation, specific antidotes, and dressings)
- Specific concerns (eg. circumferential burns to trunk or limbs, associated injuries requiring urgent definitive treatment)
- Remember AMPLE (allergies, medication, past medical history, last ate and drank, events)
- Any patient with suspected inhalation injuries *must* be assessed by an anaesthetist prior to arranging a transfer. This includes transfers to the burns unit from an on-site emergency department
- The information above should be recorded by the member of staff taking the referral; the standardized proforma in Appendix 1 may be used for this purpose.

Prior to accepting any burn for admission, the accepting clinician should liaise with the burn unit and/or the intensive care unit (ICU) to ensure that there are available beds. A useful algorithm for this process is provided in Fig. 6.1.

If an appropriate bed is not available at the closest burns unit, the burn clinician should suggest that the referrer contact the National Burns Bed Bureau (if in the UK) or the equivalent national or regional coordinating body to find the nearest available specialist burns unit bed.

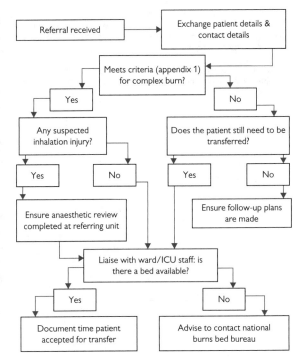

Fig. 6.1 Accepting a burns patient for admission.

Ensuring safe patient transfer

Once the decision has been made to accept the patient by a burns unit, care should be taken that the transfer is undertaken promptly and safely.

The receiving member of staff should ensure that the transfer proforma is completed, and that any pre-transfer assessments and treatments requested by them have been undertaken by the referring team (Appendix 1).

They should confirm that the patient's airway remains patent and that their physiological status has not changed since the initial referral.

Care should be taken to ensure that appropriate fluid resuscitation has been initiated and will continue at the correct rate during the transfer, and that the transferring ambulance crew has the appropriate equipment and expertise, with accompanying medical escort if indicated.

The referring team should be reminded to send copies of all medical notes, investigation results and imaging to the receiving burns unit with the patient.

The aim is to minimize the risk of the patient deteriorating en route to the burns unit, on what may be a long distance or cross-regional transfer. *Over-resuscitation is common due to over-estimation of the burn surface area. Monitor urine output during a long transfer and alter the rate of fluid administration as required.*

The priority is to get the patient to the burns unit as quickly and safely as possible, while minimizing delays and preventing cooling of the patient during the transfer.

Admitting and assessing the burns patient following transfer

Upon arriving at the burns unit, the patient should be assessed through a formal and systematic process that includes

- A specialist medical assessment (to include a complete ATLS primary and secondary survey and formal anaesthetic review of the airway and ventilation if indicated)
- Re-assessment of the burns depth and extent (including any circumferential injuries). Exposure and rolling is essential to ensure accurate TBSA
- Any routine investigations not already undertaken
- Cleaning, photography, microbiology swabs and definitive dressing of the burns wounds
- Warming of the patient if required
- Re-calculation and implementation of fluid resuscitation if required
- Treatment of any associated injuries or comorbidities
- Initiating prophylaxis for deep vein thrombosis
- Administering appropriate analgesia
- Prescribing the patient's regular medication
- Nutritional assessment and supplementation if required
- Initiating prophylaxis for stress ulceration if required
- Assessment and treatment of any drug or alcohol withdrawal needs
- Tetanus prophylaxis

Admission proforma

With frequent changeover of junior staff and cross-cover arrangements out of hours, burns units are often faced with medical staff members who may be inexperienced and unfamiliar with the unit's protocols.

Burns units should therefore consider using a proforma to help ensure that any required information is collected and that all components of the standard management plan are instituted.

A suggested admission proforma based on existing versions currently in use in the United Kingdom is available in Appendix 3.

Routine blood tests

The blood tests in Table 6.1 are recommended when a burns patient arrives on the specialist burns unit.

Table 6.1 Routine blood tests

Haematological	Biochemical
Full blood count	Urea and electrolytes
	Estimated glomerular filtration rate
Ferritin	Bicarbonate
Folate	
Vitamin B12	Magnesium
	Calcium
Coagulation screen	Zinc
	Phosphate
Group and save	Glucose
Cross-match as indicated	
	Liver function tests, including:
	Albumin
	Protein
	Globulin
	Enzymes
	Arterial blood gases if inhalation injury, and a carboxyhaemaglobin level

Predicting mortality and end of life care

Predicting mortality

Predicting mortality in burns patients is a complex and difficult process. It can be obvious from the outset; however, it is sometimes determined by the response to treatment. The decision should only be made after a multi-disciplinary discussion.

Prognostic scoring systems

- Aim to predict outcome using predictive pre-morbid and injury factors
- Limited use in clinical setting, not a replacement for clinical judgement
- Not an absolute predictor of good/poor outcome
- Good for discussions with family regarding prognosis as helpful to give figures
- Perfect scoring system has not yet been determined
- Excellent for triggering internal practice review if variance noted
- Burn-specific and general scoring systems available

Burn-specific scoring systems

Baux score – 1961

- Mortality = age + %TBSA burn
- Later modified taking into account burn depth to the prognostic burn index (PBI)
- PBI = TBSA full thickness + ½ (TBSA partial thickness) + age[1]

Abbreviated Burn Severity Index (ABSI) – 1982

- Uses five variables (gender, age, inhalational injury, TBSA, presence of Full Thickness burn)
- Power of each variable assigned a numerical value which varies according to severity
- The sum of these values is used to predict mortality[2]

Ryan Score – 1998

- Risk factors for mortality include TBSA >40%, age >60, and inhalational injury
- Scoring system based on presence of any of these three factors
- 0 = 0.3%, 1 = 3%, 2 = 33%, all three factors = 90% chance of mortality[3]

Cape Town Modified Burn Score – 1998

- Created to improve upon the Baux score
- Inhalation injury graded as mild = 1, moderate = 2, severe = 3
- Modified burn score = age + %TBSA + (20 × inhalational score)[4]

Belgian Outcome in Burn Injury (BOBI) Score – 2009

- Most recent scoring system, aimed to increase the predictive value of the Ryan score
- Subdivides patients according to age, TBSA, and presence of inhalational injury
- Sum of scores gives a prediction of mortality[5]

General non-burn scoring systems

- Acute Physiology and Chronic Health Evaluation (APACHE) score[6]
- Sepsis Related Organ Failure Assessment (SOFA)[7]
- Simplified Acute Physiology Score (SAPS)[8]

End of life care

- Despite improvements in burn care and ITU, the ultimate outcome for some is still death
- Department of Health and general Medical Council guidance aimed at standardizing end of life care
- Multidisciplinary decision needed at point of futility, and should involve the family

Principles of end of life care in burns

The principles of end of life care in burns are summarised below and in Fig. 7.1.[9]

Section 1: Initial assessment
- Physical symptom relief, eg. nausea and pain
- Spiritual care, eg. religious beliefs
- Patient/family communication
- Rationalization of unnecessary interventions
- Dressing needs, eg. odour control and comfort
- Medications are given IV due to unpredictability of the subcutaneous route in burns

Section 2: Ongoing care
- Recording of observations
- Four-hourly basis to reduce interruptions between patient and family
- Comfort goals recorded as achieved (A) or variance (V)
- If V then adjustments in care made to achieve comfort

After death care
- Contact coroner
- Contact family doctor/GP
- Minimize family distress

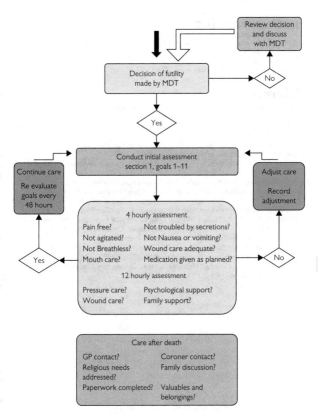

Fig. 7.1 The principles of end of life care in burns.

Reprinted from Hemington-Gorse SJ, et al. Comfort care in burns: The Burn Modified Liverpool Care Pathway (BM-LCP). *Burns* 2011:37(6):981–85, Copyright © 2011 Elsevier Ltd and ISBI, with permission from Elsevier.

Further reading

Sheppard NN, Hemington-Gorse S, Shelley B, Dziewulski P. Prognostic scoring systems in burns: a review. Burns 2011;37:1288–95.
Hemington-Gorse SJ, Clover AJP, Macdonald C, et al. Comfort care in burns: the burn modified Liverpool Care Pathway (BM-LCP). Burns 2011;37:981–85.

References

1. Baux. Contribution a l'etude du traitement local des brulures thermiques etendues. These Paris; 1961.
2. Tobiasen J, Hiebert JM, Edlich RF. The abbreviated burnseverity index. Annals of Emergency Medicine 1982;11:260–2.
3. Ryan CM, Schoenfeld DA, Thorpe WP, et al. Objective estimates of the probability of death from burn injuries. New England Journal of Medicine 1998;338:362–6.
4. Godwin, Wood. Major burns in Cape Town: a modified burns score for patient triage. Burns 1998;24:58–63.
5. Belgian Outcome in Burn Injury Study Group. Development and validation of a model for prediction of mortality in patients with acute burn injury. British Journal of Surgery 2009;96111–7.
6. Knaus WA, Zimmerman JE, Wagner DP, et al. APACHE – acute physiology and chronic health evaluation: a physiologically based classification system. Critical Care Medicine 1981;9:591–7.
7. Vincent JL, Moreno R, Takala J, Willatts S, et al. The SOFA (Sepsis-related Organ Failure Assessment) score to describe organ dysfunction/failure. On behalf of the Working Group on Sepsis-Related Problems of the European Society of Intensive Care
8. Le Gall JR, Lemeshow S, Saulnier F. A new Simplified Acute Physiology Score (SAPS II) based on a European/North American multicenter study. JAMA 1993;270:2957–63.
9. Hemington-Gorse SJ, Clover AJ, Macdonald C, et al. Comfort care in burns: the Burn Modified Liverpool Care Pathway (BM-LCP). Burns 2011;37:981–5.

Burns first aid

Importance of simple burns first aid

In the UK alone there are approximately 175,000 acute burn injuries seen by emergency services every year. Despite these numbers, there is a great variation in the way these injuries are managed prior to reaching hospital both by those providing the initial first aid and also pre-hospital medical and paramedic services.

Advances in our understanding of the pathophysiology and natural history of burn injuries have highlighted the importance of early intervention in minimizing later functional and cosmetic morbidity associated with these injuries.

Differences in beliefs and ethnic background have a large impact on the way that burns are initially dealt with, as we know that only a minority of patients presenting with burns are optimally managed before they reach hospital.

Lack of education and conflicting information about burns first aid is believed to be a major factor in the common occurrence of burnt patients presenting with a variety of domestic remedies (toothpaste, garlic, potato peel, butter, milk) being applied to their burns as first aid.

Judicious application of simple burns first aid is the first step for soft tissue preservation, improvement of outcomes, and a decrease in the need for operative management.

Steps of burns first aid

- SAFE approach
- Stop the burning process
- Cool and manage the burn wound

SAFE approach

The British Burns Association has adopted the SAFE approach acronym standing for:

- **S**hout or call for HELP
- **A**ssess the scene for dangers to rescuers or patients
- **F**ree from danger
- **E**valuate the casualty

As the first responders to burn injuries may be non-professional bystanders at the trauma scene, it is important that any individuals administering burns first aid do so in a systematic way. The initial steps of first aid should focus on ensuring that the patient and the first aider are safe and that help is sought early on. Lack of education and understanding, language barriers, and fear may all delay presentation. First aid education should therefore highlight the need to seek medical attention earlier rather than later in burn injuries.

Stop the burning process

Once the initial evaluation of the scene is complete and the first-aider is deemed safe, the priority is to halt the burning process and limit the extent of the injury to the patient. These steps should be carried out without hindering later assessment and management of the burn by application of inappropriate dressings and cleaning materials. The patient must be removed from the burning source and the burning process stopped as soon as possible. In flame burns it is advisable that the patient is prevented from running as this creates a fanning effect on the flames and may make the situation worse. In addition, the patient should be laid flat on the ground facing upwards to reduce the risk of flames involving the head and neck. Burnt clothing should be removed (unless stuck to the wounds) and jewellery taken off as this may later lead to constriction of swollen body parts. Removed clothing should be kept with the patient for later evaluation by the hospital burns team.

Cool and manage the burn wound

Cooling the burn wound

When the burning process has been stopped, it is important that the burnt area is cooled to minimise further tissue damage.

The use of clean, cool water for this purpose has the greatest evidence in the literature. Multiple studies have supported previous circumstantial evidence that immediate application of cold water (15°C) for 20 minutes to a burn injury gives the optimal result in terms of later re-epithelialization and scar result.

Cold water also has the additional proven benefits to the burnt area.
- Decrease mortality
- Pain relief
- Decreases cell damage
- Decrease skin temperature to below dangerous level
- Decreases cell metabolism in hypoxic tissue for greater cell survival
- Stabilizes vasculature
- Reduces oedema
- Improves wound healing and scar formation
- Decreases inflammatory response

It is therefore recommended that first aiders ensure that burns are irrigated with cold running water for 20 minutes.

Ice is not recommended as this may also create a thermal injury.

If this initial irrigation has not been performed, there is patchy evidence that later irrigation up to 3 hours post burn may still provide benefit. Various different agents for initial burns lavage and cooling have come and gone out of fashion over time and in different cultures.

There is little or no evidence for the benefits of anything other than cold water for initial first aid management of burns and indeed the use of substances such as oils or toothpaste can even hinder later assessment of the injuries by medical professionals.

In order to stop the burning process in chemical burns, more lengthy periods of irrigation are often required. However, exposure of some powders and other chemicals such as carbolic acid or phenol to water can worsen the injury by creating an exothermic reaction. This complicates matters generally so specific information about the causative agent should be taken with the patient to hospital with them if possible.

Managing the burn wound

Once the burn has been irrigated, it is important to cover the burn with a temporary dressing. This maintains the uncontaminated microenvironment by preventing bacterial exposure to the burn and also improves patient comfort. Clingfilm is the most widely used and appropriate temporary dressing, except in chemical burns where it may in fact worsen the injury. An alternative is a clean cool damp cloth.

It is advisable that smaller pieces of Clingfilm are placed on a wound rather than circumferentially wrapped as there is a theoretical risk of constriction with the latter. Once the burn is covered it is important to keep the patient warm by minimizing exposure. The patient should be covered and the protected burn wrapped for this purpose. Children and the elderly are at particular risk of hypothermia so this is of particular importance in these groups.

A useful mnemonic to aid in education of these basic first aid steps is **STOP**
- **S**trip hot clothes and jewellery
- **T**urn on cold tap (never use ice)—run burn under cold water for 10 minutes. Keep the rest of the patient warm.
- **O**rganise medical assistance (999/A&E/GP)
- **P**rotect burn with cling film or clean cloth (do not use dressings, fluffy cloth, creams or lotions)

Initial management by medical personnel

In the community setting, the majority of burns will first come into medical contact with either paramedic services or the patients' GP.

The key aspects of this phase of pre-hospital care are
- Basic ATLS assessment if appropriate
- Assessment of burns severity/size/depth
- Resuscitation IV fluids in large burns
- Analgesia
- History
- Early transport for definitive management

It is important that medical personnel have a good basic understanding of burns management for dealing with such patients. Recent surveys of healthcare workers have shown that health care workers in general have a limited understanding of the basics of burns care. First-aid courses with a particular focus on burns improves this basic knowledge and this should therefore be mandatory for all healthcare workers.

Basic ATLS

When a burnt patient is first assessed by paramedic or other medical service it is important that the mechanism of the burn is considered, and if appropriate, an *ATLS ABCDE* (Airways/C-spine, Breathing, Circulation, Disability, Environment) approach adopted. Any first aid steps not carried out by those first attending the patient should also be carried out if appropriate. Burns often have associated injuries, particularly if they are in the context of a house fire or motor accident, among other causes. In patients with suspected concomitant injuries, the airway should be secured, and if appropriate, the cervical spine immobilized.

In large burns and in those suspected of having inhalational injuries (for example flame burns in an enclosed space) it is essential that high flow oxygen is given via a non-rebreathing mask as soon as possible.

Assessment of burns severity/size/depth

Estimation of burn size is essential to decide if IV fluids are required.

There are several methods for calculation of burn percentage including
- The Wallace rule of nines
- The "half burnt/half not" approach (which is only generally used in pre-hospital care).
- The patients palm size (1% TBSA)
- Chart-based methods

Resuscitation IV fluids in large burns

If it is felt that the burn is greater than 10% TBSA in children or 15% in adults then cannulation should be carried out at the scene and warmed IV fluid started.

Hartmann's fluid is the recommended fluid choice. Ideally the fluid requirements should be calculated based on the Parkland formula, however, this is almost always not appropriate at the scene as the calculations will delay proceedings.

In the elderly and those with a significant cardiac history or known left ventricular failure, care should be taken not to over hydrate these patients.

Analgesia

It is also important to consider pain in acute burns, which may be considerable in some cases, particularly more superficial burns.

If the patient is cannulated, IV morphine may be given and titrated to effect, accompanied by an antiemetic.

In children, intranasal diamorphine is a suitable alternative.

Inhaled nitrous oxide may also be given but should only be used when morphine is not suitable or unavailable.

History

A concise history should be taken from the patients regarding the time and mechanism of the burn, whether the burn was in a confined space, past medical history, medications and allergies and time of the patient last ate or drank (as per ATLS guidelines).

It should also be noted, it is important to consider the possibility of non-accidental injury in all children and the elderly presenting with unusual patterns of injury or delay in presentation.

Early transport for definitive management

Once the patient is initially stabilized the patient should be delivered or transferred to either the nearest A&E or if possible, the nearest burns unit. This will depend on local protocols. Initial assessment should always aim to minimise on-scene time and deliver the patient to the appropriate medical services as soon as possible. Communication with the receiving department should be by the standard approach used nationally (age, sex, injury, ABC problems, treatment, and estimated time of arrival). Ensure that the cooling of the wound does not result in over-cooling of the patient.

Conclusion

Pre-hospital care consists of two major components:

- Basic first aid
- Later assessment and initial management by out of hospital medical services including paramedics, GPs and nurse practitioners

It is common that burns are not appropriately treated because of poor knowledge of basic burns care by non-medically trained individuals who are usually first on the scene after a burn has occurred. A solution to this problem is adoption of a simple and standard approach to burns first aid education programmes as the initial management of a burn may substantially influence the final outcome in patients with burns.

The above text summarizes the current approach to pre-hospital management and highlights the requirement for widespread education to optimize this initial phase of management in these patients.

Further reading

Greaves I, Hodgetts TJ, Porter K. (ed.) Basic life support. In Emergency care a textbook for paramedics, WB Saunders 1997; pp. 17–26.

British Burns Association first aid position statement. Available from

British Burns Association Pre-hospital Approach to Burns Patient Management: http://www.britishburnsassociation.org/pre-hospital-care

IHCD. Ambulance service basic training. Bristol: IHCD 1991.

IHCD. Ambulance service paramedic training. 3. Bristol: IHCD 1994.

Mlcak RP, Buffalo MP, Jimenez CJ. Pre hospital management, transportation and emergency care. In Herndon D (ed.) Total burn care, 4th edn. New York: Elsevier 2013.

National Association of Emergency Medical Technicians. Pre-hospital trauma life support manual 1994. Clinton, MS: NAEMT, 1994.

Weekes R. Scene approach, assessment and safety. In Greaves I, Porter K (eds) Pre-hospital medicine. The principles and practice of immediate care, London: Arnold, 1999; pp. 273–9.

Wallace HJ, O'Neill TB, Wood FM, et al. Determinants of burn first aid knowledge: cross-sectional study. Burns 39:1162–9.

Assessment of burn surface area

Initial assessment

Early, accurate assessment of the extent of a burn injury is central to successful resuscitation, and influences the mortality of burns patients. Two key elements must be assessed:

- The percentage of the total body surface area (%TBSA) burned
- The depth of burn

Remember, the TBSA burned is directly correlated with the risk of death.

Assessment of TBSA

There are a number of methods that allow the clinician to rapidly assess the area of burn. Clinicians must NOT include simple erythema in the assessment. If in doubt, gently wipe a suspicious area of burn with clean gauze, if the surface easily sloughs away it is indeed burned and must be included in TBSA. This is in contrast to areas of simple erythema that resemble sunburn and which should not be incorporated into TBSA estimations.

The palm of the hand is 1% (that of the patient, not the clinician)

This is most useful for assessing relatively small burns (<10% TBSA) that may be patchy such as scald injury in a child. It becomes less accurate in assessing large areas of burn injury.

Wallace rule of nines

This method divides the body into sections of 9%, or multiples thereof (see Table 9.1).

This technique is best suited for larger burns in adult patients. The proportions are altered in children where the head comprises a relatively higher surface area (and the limbs less so) and thus can lead to an inaccurate assessment of burn size.

Lund and Browder chart

This current "gold standard" of TBSA assessment was devised in 1940, and is similar to the Wallace rule of nines with further refinement. In particular, paediatric patients are more reliably assessed with clearly tabulated guides to age related changes in surface area (see Fig. 9.1).

In a large burn, it may be simpler to estimate the unburned area and subtract it from 100%.

Estimation of hand surface area, and small burns

The hand is a common site of burn injury, and the area involved varies considerably. A simple method of estimation is to express the area involved in terms of the patient's thumbprint area (T) (Table 9.2), which can also be used to estimate small burns (<1% TBSA) elsewhere in the body.

- Calculation of % surface area = number of thumbprints ÷ 30
- One thumbprint (T) = 1/30th of 1% = 0.033% TBSA
  - 3T burn = 0.1% TBSA

Table 9.1 Rule of nines

Area	% TBSA
Head	9
Each upper limb	9
Each lower limb	18
Front of trunk	18
Back of trunk	18
Perineum	1

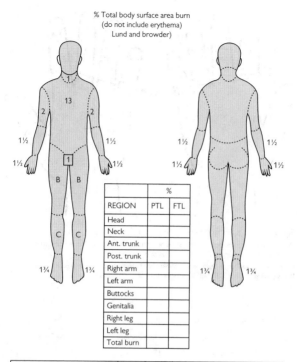

% Total body surface area burn
(do not include erythema)
Lund and browder)

	%	
REGION	PTL	FTL
Head		
Neck		
Ant. trunk		
Post. trunk		
Right arm		
Left arm		
Buttocks		
Genitalia		
Right leg		
Left leg		
Total burn		

AREA	Age 0	1	5	10	15	Adult
A-1½ OF HEAD	9½	8½	6½	5½	4½	3½
B-1½ OF ONE HEAD	2¾	3¼	4	4½	4½	4¾
C-½ OF ONE LOWER LEG	2½	2½	2¾	3	3¼	3½

Fig. 9.1 Lund and Browder Chart.

Reproduced from Smith J, Greaves I, Porter KM (eds). *Oxford desk reference: major trauma*, Figure 22.7, Copyright © Oxford University Press 2007, with permission from Oxford University Press.

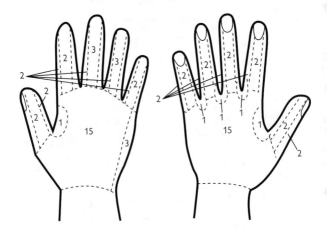

Fig. 9.2 Hand burns surface area: a rule of thumb.

Diagram of surface areas of the hand, showing estimated thumbprint (T) areas on each surface, including web spaces and radial/ulnar surfaces of digits.

Reproduced from Dargan D, Mandal A, Shokrollahi K. Hand burns surface area: a rule of thumb. Burns (in press, March 2018) with permission from Elsevier.

Table 9.2 Rule of thumb

Surface areas of the hand	Thumbprints (T)	% TBSA
Palm (excluding digits)	15	0.5
Dorsum (excluding digits)	15	0.5
Radial, ulnar palmar and dorsal aspects of each digit (20 surfaces)	2 on each surface, on each digit* (total 42)	**0.066**(1.4)
First web space	2	0.066
2nd, 3rd, 4th web spaces	1 on each space (total 3)	**0.033**(0.1)
Ulnar border of palm	3	0.1
Whole hand	80	2.66

*Volar surface of ring and middle finger 3T each.

Newer techniques

Technologies such as smartphone apps and similar strategies have been employed successfully to give accurate and rapid assessments with less margins of error, such as the validated Mersey Burns App which can be used as an app or simply via the weblink on any computer or smart device, www.merseyburns.com.

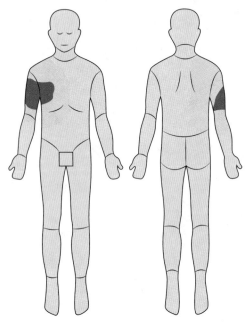

Fig. 9.3 Mersey Burns App image of burns to chest, back and right upper limb. Full thickness areas are in red, partial thickness in pink. TBSA Estimated at 15.5% using the website, www.merseyburns.com.

Reproduced with permission from Mersey Burns.

Further reading

Barnes J, Duffy A, Hamnett N, et al. The Mersey Burns App: evolving a model of validation. Emergency Medicine Journal 2015;32:637–41.

Dargan D, Mandal A, Shokrollahi K. Hand burns surface area: a rule of thumb. Burns 2018;44:1346–51.

Burn depth assessment

Introduction to burn depth assessment

Why burn depth assessment?

Burn depth assessment is essential for the planning of care and prevention of scar formation. This however is a difficult task due to the evolving nature of burns. If a deep burn is not surgically excised it has the potential to become colonized with bacteria, increasing morbidity and potentially mortality. Hypertrophic scarring becomes more likely the longer the burn wound is left, therefore it is important to assess depth as deeper burns will take longer to heal. Burns which are likely to take longer than 2 weeks to heal in children and 3 weeks for adults should be considered for intervention as it is after these time frames that the risks of hypertrophic scarring becomes significant.

Difficulties with burn assessments

Jackson described three zones of a burn wound. These are:

- Zone of coagulation: area of necrosis and irreversible tissue destruction
- Zone of stasis: adjacent to the zone of coagulation which describes at-risk tissue. This tissue has decreased tissue perfusion, which without optimal care will progress to necrosis. It is within this area where deepening of burns occurs over 48 hours
- Zone of hyperaemia: this is the tissue surrounding the zone of stasis in which inflammatory mediators cause widespread dilatation of blood vessels, clinically, it has the appearance of erythema. After the acute phase this zone returns to normal perfusion

It is the evolution of the zone of stasis into the zone of coagulation which can deepen the burn wound and cause difficulties with assessing wound depth.

There are various factors which influence conversion of zones, and hence increased burn depth. This is usually the result of a reduction in the microcirculation due to changes in blood pressure, localized oedema or thrombosis, which leads to tissue hypoxia.

If the wound is not debrided it is difficult to assess the underlying skin and depth. Usually burn wounds are not homogenous but a mixed pattern, thereby complicating assessment.

In an electrical burn the current travels through the body, and creates entry and exit wounds. Between these two points underlying tissue damage can result from the heat generated by the current. This damage will not be visible by inspecting the skin only.

Classification

There are many different ways to describe burn depth. Here we will describe it by histological depth.

Epidermal: first-degree burns/erythema

The epidermal burns are erythematous only. They appear as pink, painful areas which blanch with light pressure and don't form blisters. These are not counted as true burns and as such not included in the estimation of total body surface area. These will heal over a couple of days by the shedding of the outer layers of the epidermis.

Superficial partial thickness: second-degree burns (2a)/superficial dermal burns

These involve all of the epidermis and the superficial part of the dermis, leaving the deeper part of the dermis intact. These will usually have intact or ruptured blisters, leaving the dermis exposed, shiny, oozy and pink. The wound will have a capillary refill of less than 2 seconds and become very painful. Rubbing with a finger may shear off the epidermis. These will usually heal within 3 weeks and leave no scarring. However, there may be discoloration in pigmented skin and this may take up to 2–3 years to resolve. They heal by migration of keratinocytes from the base of the burn wound –these cells travel up from keratinocyte reserves surrounding adnexal structures, which originate deeper than the level of burn.

Deep partial thickness: second-degree (2b)/deep dermal

This involves all of the epidermis, superficial dermis, and mid-dermis.
  They appear as a dark shade of red (cherry red) due to the thrombosed blood in the dermal capillaries. This red staining is fixed and will not blanch with pressure. Because the deeper adnexal structures are damaged the reserve of keratinocytes are also lost. This means relying on migration of the cells from the wound edge and results in healing taking more than 3 weeks.

Full thickness: third-degree/subdermal

This involves all layers of the epidermis and dermis. Characteristically they have a leathery eschar which is either white or black (if carbonized) and are insensate as the sensory nerve endings have been damaged. They heal by wound contraction and migration of keratinocytes from the wound's edge.
  Circumferential full thickness burns can impair limb circulation and chest wall expansion by acting as a restrictive band. Re-establishment may require escharotomies.

Catastrophic: Fourth-degree burns

This term is used to describe full thickness burns which have also damaged underlying structures (bone, cartilage, organs/brain, etc.).

Modalities to assess burns

There are many different modalities to assess burn depth.

Clinical

This relies on burnt skin colour, sensation, appearance, blanching, and blister formation.

Accuracy—depends on the experience of the clinician but can vary between 50% and 80%, with indeterminate dermal burns being the most difficult to assess. Clinical assessment is highly accurate in very superficial and very deep burns and these do not require additional technological methods. Owing to the evolving nature of burn wounds they should be reassessed after 48 hours to see if there has been any burn depth progression. Accuracy does not vary between 2 and 5 days however between 5 and 14 days assessment becomes difficult due to the decrease in inflammatory response and the use of topical agents.

Useful adjuncts

Blanching

Pressing on the burn to see the colour disappear and turn white. This is caused by the occlusion and emptying of the capillaries. In deeper burns the small capillaries have been burnt and thrombosed, leading to fixed staining.

Hair follicles

Hair follicles lie in the deeper part of the dermis. Hairs that are easily dislodged by a small tug with forceps indicate a deeper dermal burn.

Clarke's sign

Sweat glands originate deep in the dermis and protrude through the epidermal layer, resulting in sweat emerging from the skin. Clarke's sign says that when there is sweating of the burn this indicates a more superficial burn as this indicates the sweat glands are not damaged.

Pinprick tests

Pinprick tests can be a good discriminator between superficial and deep burns in a number of ways. Pain discriminates well between superficial (painful) and deep (painless to insensate) burns. The briskness or absence of bleeding to pinprick is also a good discriminator as delayed or absent bleeding would signify a deeper burn.

"Test shave" in theatre

Very thin tangential excision of the deepest part of an intermediate depth burn can be valuable. Adjunctive debridement techniques such as "VersaJet" hydro-debridement can be used in a similar way.

Remembered by some as "red is dead", "White is alright".

Clinical assessment

Table 10.1 provides an overview of the clinical assessment for burns.

Table 10.1 Clinical assessment table for burns

Classification	Degree	Layer of skin involved	Examples	Appearance	Time to heal	Sensation	Blanching	Bleeding
Superficial	1st degree	Epidermis	Sunburn	Redness but not blistered	3–4 days kerationcytes regenerate damage	Highly sensitive/ painful	Yes	Brisk
Superficial Partial Thickness	2nd degree (2a)	Epidermis+ Papillary Dermis	Scald	Red/Blistered Moist	2–3 weeks	Sensitive/ painful	Yes	Brisk
Deep partial thickness (deep dermal)	2nd degree (2b)	Epidermis + Reticular dermis	Contact	Dark shade of red	>3 weeks	Sensation decreased	Fixed Staining	Slow
Full thickness	3rd Degree	All layers involved	Flame	White/Black Leathery	Never unless very small	Absent	Non blanching	Absent
Catastrophic	4th degree	Through skin and involves underlying structures	Flame	White/black Leathery	Never	Absent	Non blanching	Absent

Technology

There are three main areas in which technology is being used in burns depth assessment. These are:

- Tissue perfusion
- Surface colour
- Structural analysis

Extremely important is the concept that **the burn wound is dynamic not static** and assessment at one point in time should be interpreted with this in mind. There remain considerable differences of opinion in regard to the role of clinical vs. objective measures of burn depth assessment and some believe that NICE guidelines in favour of laser Doppler assessments have over-reached.

Tissue perfusion

It is assumed that a deeper burn will correlate with a lower blood perfusion due to blood vessels either being destroyed or thrombosed. Clinically we judge this by the blanching of the skin.

The problem with all tissue perfusion measurement is that a number of other factors can effect tissue perfusion. These include:

- Hypothermia
- Room temperature
- Vasoconstructive drugs
- Tourniquets
- Hypovolaemia
- Respiratory rate
- Patient's emotional state

Laser Doppler

Laser Doppler technology uses the measurement in alteration in light to measure the velocity and number of moving particles.

Laser Doppler flowmetry

Initially laser dopplers were introduced in 1975 and required contact with the burn wound – this is known as laser Doppler flowmetry (LDF). This method was proven to be 70-100% accurate in predicting healing within 21 days and 93–100% accurate in predicting failure to heal.

However, a number of problems were identified with the method, which included:

- Contact needed with burn wound, leading to increased infection risk and pain
- Pressure with probe, leading to occlusion and artificial results
- Only a small area could be scanned (1 mm area)

Laser Doppler imager

Owing to the problems of the LDF requiring contact with the patient laser Doppler imagers (LDIs) were introduced in the 1990s. LDIs could scan a larger area and used a non-touch technique. The laser typically penetrates 1–2 mm. Before 48 hours accuracy in indeterminate depths is less than 80% and this compares to a 60–70% clinical accuracy. They have therefore been recommended for scanning between 2–5 days.

NICE guidelines (2011) recommend LDI use for all intermediate depth burn wounds. However, many burns surgeons feel that this guidance came prematurely and assessment and treatment of intermediate depth burns is both controversial and varied amongst burns surgeons.

Depending on the make and local hospital policies safety goggles may need to be worn.

There are two types of commercially available LDIs:
- Scanning LDI
  - A laser is reflected onto the skin by moving mirrors to produce a scan of the area. Reflected light from the skin is then mirrored back to the photodiodes
- Speckle LDI
  - The laser source hits the surface of the skin and forms a speckle pattern. This reflects the coherence of the source and the microcirculation of the skin. The pattern is received over a time period and relayed to the screen

Interpretation

Laser dopplers measure inflammatory response therefore a high reading would be expected in superficial burns.

Unburnt skin has low blood flow and therefore will appear to look like a deep burn.

As the LDI depends on blood flow they are only accurate before the inflammatory phase of the burn declines and the dermal circulation stabilizes. This occurs between 48 hours and 5 days.

The results of the machines are recorded in perfusion units. Traditionally these perfusion units are scaled against healing times (see Table 10.2)

LDI problems

Movement of the patient or machine, however small, gives an inaccurate image of perfusion. Therefore a deep burn can appear more superficial, because the machine will analyse the movement as blood flow and thereby lead to misdiagnosis.

Undebrided, tattooed, and darker pigmented skins effect the penetration of the laser and therefore will give low readings.

Table 10.2 Interpreting laser Doppler results

Inflammatory response/velocity of red blood cells	LDI colour	Potential healing time
High	Red	<14 days
Medium	Yellow	14–21
Same as unburnt skin or lower	Blue	>21

Reproduced from Pape et al. (2012) Burn wound healing time assessed by laser Doppler imaging (LDI). Part 1: Derivation of a dedicated colour code for image interpretation Burns 38(2):187–94 with permission from Elsevier

Angle artefact

The LDI must be parallel to the area skin to be scanned to get the maximum recording of the reflected light. If this angle changes you do not get the full reflection of the laser, leading to an lower, inaccurate reading. This can happen on small areas (eg. fingers), where a body part curves away (eg. flank, arm, leg), or if the laser is not set up correctly.

- Different areas of the body have different perfusions therefore an area may be misdiagnosed
- Topical agents disrupt LDI readings as they form a barrier to laser penetrance
- Distance measured can also effect readings

Other measures of tissue perfusion

- Injection techniques of either radioactive isotopes or dyes. Presence would imply good perfusion and a superficial burn. However these are invasive, expensive and not readily available.
- Video microscopy
  - Uses a visual evaluation of vessel integrity
- Thermography
  - It is a non-contact technique which uses infrared radiation produced by the skin to assess burn depth. However environmental factors can sometimes dramatically effect readings. Progress continues to be made in this area.
  - LDI is very expensive, and after a wave of purchasing and enthusiasm, some units no longer use the equipment in favour of clinical assessments

Surface colour

Part of a clinical assessment is the colour of the wound bed, which can indicate the burn depth. Two scientific ways exist of conducting this are photography and spectrophotometry.

- Photography is increasing in popularity due to the increase in telemedicine usage. In obvious superficial and deep burns it is purported to have a 90% accuracy. However without the ability to test blanching, etc., it is of questionable use in difficult to determine wounds. This does however facilitate the storage of images
- Spectrophotometry. This judges the wound surface colour by sending light from a spectrometer and the reflected light intensity is assessed by the photometer
- Photography and telemedicine with an experienced eye can be surprisingly accurate

Structural analysis

The gold standard is considered to be histological analysis by punch biopsy. However for obvious reasons this is confined mostly to a research environment. This is due to the fact they only show the area biopsied, processing can take several days, needing expert knowledge and can leave additional scarring.

Ultrasound at high frequencies has been shown to be of some use however it requires contact with the burn and is difficult to interpret.

Further reading

Hoeksema H, Baker RD, Holland AJ, et al. A new, fast LDI for assessment of burns: a multi-centre clinical evaluation. Burns 2014;40:1274–82.

Javed M, Shokrollahi K. VACUETTE(®) for burn depth assessment—a simple and novel alternative use for a ubiquitous phlebotomy device. Burns 2012;38:1084–5.

Hop MJ, Moues CM, Bogomolova K, et al. Photographic assessment of burn size and depth: reliability and validity. Journal of Wound Care 2014;23:144–5, 148–52.

Shokrollahi K, Sayed M, Dickson W, Potokar T. Mobile phones for the assessment of burns: we have the technology. Emergency Medicine Journal 2007;24:753–5.

Fluid resuscitation in burns

Introduction to fluid resuscitation in burns

Burns injury demands fluid resuscitation when total body surface area (TBSA) exceeds 15% in adults and 10% in children.

There are two key mechanisms underlying this:

- A large volume of fluid is lost from the wound when the integrity of the epidermis is lost. The greatest loss is in the first 12 hours post burn
- Inflammatory mediators are released into the wound causing vasodilation. This process becomes systemic with burns >20% resulting in intravascular hypovolaemia. The altered capillary permeability that drives this tends to recover from 36 hours post burn

Full thickness burns develop three areas zones of decreasing injury (Jackson's burn wound model):

- Central zone of coagulative necrosis
- Intermediate zone of stasis of blood flow
- Outer zone of vasodilation and hyperaemia

The primary function of fluid resuscitation is to

- Prevent burn shock by giving adequate fluid without overloading the vascular system or causing excessive oedema
- Maintain circulatory volume in the face of losses due to the burn—this is essential for cardiac output, renal perfusion and tissue perfusion
- Provide metabolic water
- Maintain tissue perfusion to the zone of stasis and prevent the burn from deepening

With limited physiological reserve resuscitation must commence in children >10% TBSA and be accompanied by additional background fluid support.

Inhalation injury further increases fluid requirement and can represent up to an additional 20% TBSA.

There is no clear evidence to favour one resuscitation fluid over another, but most units use easily accessible crystalloid such as Hartmann's solution (Parkland).

Albumin is also often used via a different protocol (Muir and Barclay).

The crystalloid vs. colloid debate continues.

Burn Area Calculation

Do not include simple erythema

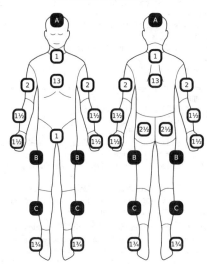

Age	0	1	5	10	15	Adult
A	9½	8½	6½	5½	4½	3½
B	2¾	3¼	4	4½	4½	4¾
C	2½	2½	2¾	3	3¼	3½

www.merseyburns.com

Calculation of fluid requirement

Parkland formula (1968)

This is the most commonly used and often recommended regimen in practice today.

Three key pieces of information are needed to commence appropriate resuscitation fluids.

- TBSA (see diagram on inside cover to aid calculation)
- Time of burn injury
- Weight of patient

The Parkland formula for the total fluid requirement in **24 hours** following burn injury is as follows:

- 4 mL × TBSA (%) × body weight (kg)
- 50% given in first 8 hours
- 50% given in next 16 hours
  - Children receive maintenance fluid (4% glucose in one-quarter or one-fifth saline) in addition, at an hourly rate of:
  - 4 mL/kg for the first 10 kg of body weight plus
  - 2 mL/kg for the second 10 kg of body weight plus
  - 1 mL/kg for >20 kg of body weight
- For accuracy, subtract any amount of fluid already given from the requirements for the first 8 hours

Beware hyponatraemia in children and use background fluids of 5% dextrose in half-normal saline if transfer is delayed >12 hours.

- Fluids should run through two large bore IV cannulae ideally inserted through non-burnt skin. Intraosseus infusion may be needed in children.
- Worked example:
  - 10 kg child suffers 20% TBSA and arrives in department 2 hours following injury
  - Resuscitation requirement as per Parkland formula
  - 4 × 10 × 20 = 800 mL in 24 hours
  - Burn was 2 hours ago, therefore fluid for first 8-hour time period must go through in 6 hours
  - Thus 800/2 = 400 mL over 6 hours, ie. **66 mL per hour for 6 hours**
  - Followed by 400 mL over 16 hours, ie. 25 mL per hour for next 16 hours Hartmann's solution
  - PLUS maintenance 4 × 10 = 1000 mL, ie. 40 mL per hour 4% glucose in one-quarter normal saline

Muir and Barclay resuscitation protocol (1962)

Estimates the amount of colloid (5% human albumin solution) that needs to be administered during the first 36 hours after a major burn.

It divides up the total time into six periods of varying duration, each requiring the same volume of fluid.

- %TBSA × body weight (kg) × 0.5 = volume (mL) in each period
- 1st/2nd/3rd periods—4 hourly
- 4th/5th periods—6 hourly
- 6th period—12 hourly

When using this formula, maintenance fluid is also required.
- Combination resuscitation regimes are often used: Hartmann's for 8 hours and switch to albumin for the remaining time

Monitoring response to resuscitation

The most straightforward and reliable technique to assess adequacy is via urine output (UOP) thus demanding catheterization for patients with large burns.
- Adults 0.5 mL/kg/h. This equates to 30–50 mL per hour
- Children <30 kg 1.0 mL/kg/h

This urine output reflects adequate renal perfusion and will alert the clinician to over resuscitation if UOP is excessive, and poor tissue perfusion with associated consequences if UOP is low.

Developing acidosis can reflect hypoperfusion of tissues and under resuscitation, but may also indicate the need for, or inadequacy of, escharotomy.

It is essential to monitor serum electrolytes following resuscitation. A dilutional hyponatraemia is common and hyperkalaemia seen following electrocution.

Myoglobinuria

Tissue injury associated with electrocution, blunt trauma, or ischaemia results in the release of myoglobin and haemoglobin into the circulation. Deposition in the proximal tubules of the kidney will cause acute renal failure. The urine is typically coloured brown or orange.

Treatment

- Increase UOP to 1–2 mL/kg/h
- Mannitol 12.5 g/L resuscitation fluid
- Sodium bicarbonate 25 meq/L resuscitation fluid

Important points

- Do not put too much emphasis on fluid calculation and instead prioritize (1) transfer of patients to burns services, (2) keeping the patient warm, which is critical, (3) analgesia
- Patients are often over-resuscitated. Aim for an accurate assessment of burn and sensible fluids until they reach specialist care
- Various technological solutions exist to facilitate calculation of burn surface area and fluid resuscitation such as the Mersey Burns iPhone/iPad App, which can be accessed and used from any computer or smart device through the internet if the app is not available via www.merseyburns.com

Further reading

Alvarado R, Chung KK, Cancio LC, Wolf SE. Burn resuscitation. Burns 2009;35:41–4.

Hunter JE, Drew PJ, Potokar TS, et al. Albumin resuscitation in burns: a hybrid regime to mitigate fluid creep. Scars, Burns & Healing 2016;22;2:2059513116642083.

Tricklebank S. Modern trends in fluid therapy for burns. Burns 2009;35:7–67.

Escharotomies

Background of escharotomies

Following a significant thermal or electrical injury, tissues beneath the skin swell through fluid loss into the interstitial space. The increase in extravascular fluid together with the inelastic nature of the overlying burned skin compound to increase pressure within the affected limb. This increase in pressure can compromise the vascular supply distally in an affected limb or increase ventilatory pressures in those with circumferential burns of the chest and abdomen. This chapter will give guidance on when and how to perform escharotomies; however, the final decision is usually based on experience and clinical judgement.

Indications of escharotomies

- Circumferential burns of extremities that develop signs of inadequate perfusion (cool to touch, reduced pulse oximetry)
- Circumferential burns of chest and abdomen that develop ventilatory compromise or abdominal compartment syndrome
- Absence of pulse on Doppler distal to injury (presence of a pulse doesn't rule out need for escharotomy
- Compartment pressure >30 mmHg or within 30 mmHg of systolic BP. *Note—escharotomies will not treat true compartment syndrome, which will require fasciotomies*

Principles of escharotomies

- Electrocautery may be preferred to scalpel in general although some prefer scalpel especially for the digits
- Full thickness incisions through burned skin to subcutaneous tissues
- Longitudinal incisions to avoid injury to underlying neurovascular structures, with the limbs in the anatomical position
- Aim to commence and end incision within normal skin, preferably 1–2 cm from the edge of the burn
- If you are cutting through long lengths of unburned skin, reflect on the necessity or location of the escharotomy
- Experienced surgeons may deviate from 'traditional' lines of escharotomy in preference for the deepest area of burn and incise the fascia to allow assessment of any need for formal fasciotomy

Specifics of escharotomies

Please see the figures for details of regional escharotomies.

Upper limb

- Longitudinal incision along both radial and ulnar aspect of upper extremity (Fig. 12.1)
- Pass anterior to the medial epicondyle (avoid ulnar nerve injury)
- Continue incisions into hand overlying hypothenar and thenar eminence
- Dorsal hand escharotomies overlying the 2nd and 4th metacarpals can be linked to ulnar escharotomy at wrist (Fig. 12.2)
- Digital escharotomies can reduce necrosis and should be made between the neurovascular bundle and the extensors, avoiding both structures on the radial border of the thumb and ulnar border of all other digits (Fig. 12.3)

Lower limb

- Longitudinal incision along both medial and lateral aspect of lower extremity
- Pass anterior to the fibula head (avoid common peroneal nerve injury)

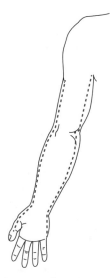

Fig. 12.1 Markings for escharotomies of upper limb. Avoid injury to ulnar nerve by passing anterior to the medial epicondyle.

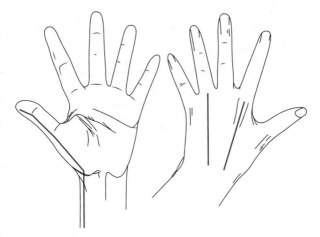

Fig. 12.2 Markings for escharotomies of thumb (continuation of radial forearm escharotomy), dorsal markings for escharotomy.

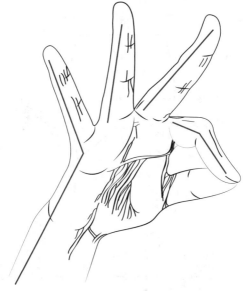

Fig. 12.3 Markings for escharotomies of digits—ulnar border of digits 2–5.

Chest and abdomen

- Join all incisions to allow a "breast plate" of tissue to move and reduce ventilatory pressures (Fig. 12.4)
- Superior incision—transverse incision inferior to the clavicles
- Longitudinal incision—along anterior axillary lines bilaterally (allow continuation along lateral borders of abdomen to decompress, if necessary)
- Inferior incision—along inferior border of costal margin
- Abdominal compartment syndrome is not infrequent and there should be a relatively low threshold for release of the abdomen as well. This is even more important in children as abdominal restriction compromises ventilation

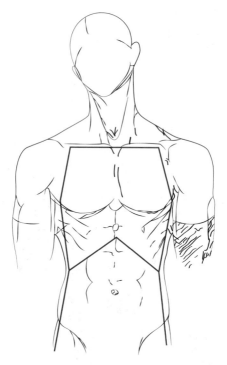

Fig. 12.4 Markings for escharotomies of chest and abdomen. Superior incision below clavicles, longitudinal incision along anterior axillary line, and inferior incision at the inferior border of the costal margin. Continuation of longitudinal incision shown to allow release of abdomen.

Practical points to consider

- Local anaesthetic if patient not sedated (lignocaine with adrenaline 1%)
- Maximum dose 7 mg/kg
- Maximum dose for 70 kg patient = 49 mL
- Dry the tissues and then use a sterile pen to mark the line that will be infiltrated with local anaesthetic
- Anatomical position
- Cutting diathermy
- Swabs/gauze ready
- Dressings: alginate dressing to assist haemostasis
- Monitor for postoperative bleeding

Fasciotomy

Preferably carried out within 6 hours of the initial injury. The indications are similar to escharotomy; however, in the case of electrical injury or exceptionally deep circumferential thermal injury a fasciotomy is preferred. The typical signs of compartment syndrome (pain, pallor, paraesthesia, paralysis, and pulselessness) are sometimes difficult to assess in the acute stages after admission due to mechanical ventilation and sedation. Loss of pulse is a late finding in compartment syndrome. However, if possible, these should be checked regularly as any changes can give rise to the need for intervention.

Upper limbs

Forearm

Dorsal

Incision is longitudinal and may be linked to the dorsal hand incisions as per the diagram. It is important to release all compartments in the hand (Fig. 12.5).

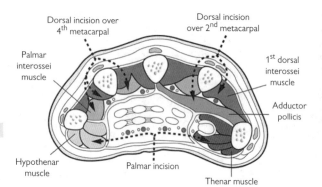

Fig. 12.5 Fasciotomies of the hand showing release of dorsal and palmar interossei. Lateral and medial incisions to release thenar and hypothenar muscles respectively.

Adapted from Green DP, et al. (eds). Green's operative hand surgery, 5th edn. Philadelphia, PA: Churchill Livingstone, Copyright © 2005, with permission from Elsevier.

Volar

Use an 'S'-shaped skin incision (Fig. 12.6).
- Starting point: between the hypothenar and thenar eminences
- Wrist and distal forearm: decompress the carpal tunnel ± Guyon's canal
- Turn incision to ulnar aspect of wrist and continue along the ulnar border of the distal forearm
- Mid-forearm: turn the incision to the radial side of the forearm and then return to the ulnar border radial to the medial epicondyle

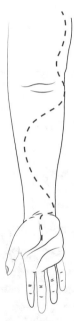

Fig. 12.6 Markings for fasciotomy of the upper limb.

Adapted from Green DP, et al. (eds). Green's operative hand surgery, 5th edn. Philadelphia, PA: Churchill Livingstone. Copyright © 2005, with permission from Elsevier.

Proximal forearm and arm

Passing volar to the medial epicondyle the incision then passes proximally into the arm along the medial border.

Aims
- Decompression of medial and ulnar nerves
- Decompression of superficial and deep compartments of forearm
- Exposure and adequate coverage of the median nerve
- Protection of cutaneous nerves and preservation of as many cutaneous veins as possible

Pitfalls
Inadequate decompression of compartments of the hand resulting in necrosis of intrinsic muscles.

Lower limb

Although the skin incision is the similar for an escharotomy and fasciotomy below the knee, the markings for the latter in an adult are approximately two fingerbreadths either side of the subcutaneous border of the tibia (Fig. 12.7).

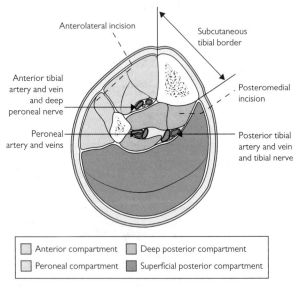

Fig. 12.7 Cross-section of the leg showing the release of all four compartments. Here we see entry into the anterior compartment and then subsequent release of the lateral compartment.

Anterior incision

Through the skin and fascia into the anterior compartment. The dissection should then be carried laterally and through the intermuscular septum into the lateral compartment.

Medial incision

Through the skin and fascia into the superficial posterior compartment, the Soleus muscle then needs to be dissected free of the medial border of the tibia allowing continued dissection through the posterior intermuscular septum in order to decompress the deep posterior compartment.

The importance of decompressing all four compartments completely cannot be over expressed. Inadequate decompression results in significant morbidity and occasionally amputation.

Thigh fasciotomies can be continuous with the incisions below the knee. The medial incision will allow decompression of the medial compartment of the thigh. The lateral incision will allow direct access and decompression of the anterior compartment from which the posterior compartment of the thigh can be easily accessed (Fig. 12.8).

Pitfalls

Beware of concealed compartment syndrome within the thigh (pain on passive extension/flexion at knee) prophylactic escharotomy/fasciotomy is low risk to prevent significant risk of distal loss of function.

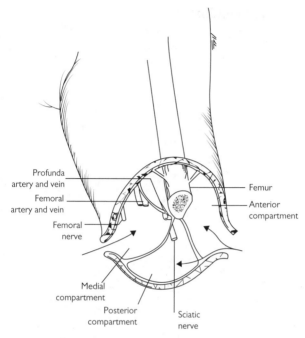

Fig. 12.8 Cross-section of the thigh showing medial and lateral fasciotomies.

Reprinted from Velmahos GC, et al. Vascular trauma and compartment syndromes. Surgical Clinics of North America 2002;82(1):125–41. Copyright © 2002 W.B. Saunders Company, with permission from Elsevier.

Further reading

Orgill DP, Piccolo N. Escharotomy and decompressive therapies in burns. Journal of Burn Care & Research 2009;30:759–68.
Velmahos GC, Toutouzas KG. Vascular trauma and compartment syndromes. Surgical clinics of North America 2002;82:125–41.

Critical care of burns patients

Definition of critical care of burns patients

The management of critically ill burns patients requires close collaboration between burns surgeons, critical care physicians, microbiologists, pharmacists, and physiotherapists in order to optimize survival of such patients. Patients with burn injury should be admitted to a Critical Care with burns expertise for joint Critical Care/Burns team management in the following circumstances:

• Inhalational injury requiring mechanical ventilation
• Extensive head/neck/chest burns requiring mechanical ventilation
• Requirement for extensive burns surgery
• Management of acute renal failure due to rhabdomyolysis

Survival of critically ill patients in general has continuously improved following the application of evidenced-based treatments, especially mechanical ventilation and these treatments should be considered for all burns patients.

Airway

The endotracheal tube in a patient with burns must be left uncut to accommodate facial swelling.

Inhalational injury

- Suspected from the history and examination
- Look for evidence of nasal hair singing, soot in oropharynx, hoarse voice
- Chest X-ray is poor at predicting the presence of inhalational injury
- Bronchoscopy has a major role in the diagnosis of inhalational injury
- Perform bronchoscopy as soon as the patient is admitted to the critical care unit
- Bronchoscopy findings may include soot deposits, erythema, mucosal oedema, mucosal ulceration and incidental presence of pneumonia
- Lavage of lungs with up to 250 mL of 0.9% sodium chloride will help to remove soot plaques

Tracheostomy

For patients who require ventilatory support or airway protection for a considerable time then a temporary tracheostomy is often required.

Benefits

- Much less irritant than oral endotracheal tube
- Patient can be awake and mechanically ventilated without the need for sedatives
- Permits patient communication, eating and earlier mobilization
- Percutaneous technique with bronchoscopic control can be performed on intensive care unit
- Relatively safe procedure

Risks

- Presence of burns around the neck or abnormal distorted anatomy may mean that a surgical tracheostomy is required
- Despite several recent trials, there is no current evidence between an early versus later tracheostomy in terms of mortality or morbidity
- Haemorrhage during procedure
- Infection around tracheostomy site
- Scarring

Breathing

Mechanical ventilation of the critically ill burns patient will be required for patients with:
• Traumatic airway injuries from explosion
• Extensive burns to the chest and neck resulting in ventilatory failure
• Injury to the lungs from inhalation of smoke, hot gases or blast injury
• Postoperative care following major burns surgery

Patients with severe burns and inhalational/blast injuries are at risk of acute respiratory distress syndrome (ARDS) and it is essential that meticulous care is applied to ventilatory strategies in order to minimize further lung damage.

ARDS

• Characterized by bilateral infiltrates on a chest X-ray with severe hypoxaemia and the absence of cardiogenic pulmonary oedema
• The mortality of patients at risk of or with ARDS is significantly reduced by a mechanical ventilation strategy using low tidal volumes (6 mL/kg based upon ideal body weight)
• Airway pressures should be kept below 30 cmH$_2$O to avoid barotrauma
• Ideal body weight is calculated using a standard height-based algorithm
• Fluid overload must be avoided

Weaning from mechanical ventilation

The ability for patients to wean from mechanical ventilation should be assessed daily when the following conditions are met:
• Fraction of inspired oxygen (FiO$_2$) 0.5 or less
• Resolution of underlying pathology, eg. pneumonia
• Decreasing requirement for vasopressors
• Resolution of pyrexia

If the patient is sedated, these should be stopped and the patient allowed to waken so that they can breathe using a spontaneous breathing mode. A spontaneous breathing trial should be undertaken using the following techniques:
• Spontaneous breathing via a 'T-piece'
• Spontaneous breathing with a CPAP circuit
• Pressure support ventilation with a Pressure support of 7 cmH$_2$O

If after 30 minutes the patient is comfortable, able to cough, minimal secretions, and obey commands, then a trial of extubation should be considered. Measurement of f/TV (where f is the patient's spontaneous breathing rate and TV is the tidal volume in litres) helps to predict weaning success: f/TV <105 predicts success.

Circulation

The use of a thermodilution catheter, eg. PiCCO or Lidco may assist by measuring the patient preload, contractility and afterload. Following adequate filling, inotropic/vasopressors drugs may be required to maintain an adequate mean arterial pressure (MAP) to ensure vital organs are perfused sufficiently.

Agents include

- Noradrenaline-alpha and beta agonist, primarily increases afterload, eg. in septic shock
- Adrenaline—alpha and beta agonist
- Dobutamine—beta agonist
- Dopexamine—inotrope with effects on splanchnic circulation and renal blood flow

Sedation and analgesia

Common sedatives for mechanically ventilated burns patients include propofol and midazolam. Ketamine is a useful sedative for burns dressing changes.

Patients should have a daily sedation 'hold' whereby the sedation is temporarily discontinued to see if they actually need ongoing—the evidence shows that sedation holds lead to a significant reduction in the duration of mechanical ventilation.

Sedation advantages

- Allows patient to tolerate endotracheal tube
- Suppresses patient's natural respiratory drive—avoids 'fighting the ventilator'
- Facilitates nursing care such as burns dressing changes
- Permits painful procedures to be done

Disadvantages

- Associated with nightmares and hallucinations
- Accumulation of metabolites leading to over sedation
- Hypotension as a side effect

Analgesia may be given in the form of intravenous morphine but the disadvantage of morphine is that it accumulates. Alternative analgesics include alfentanil (a short-acting synthetic opioid) and remifentanil (an ultra-short-acting opioid which may permit patients to be awake while intubated and ventilated).

Exposure

Critically ill patients with burns should be nursed in a warm environment to avoid hypothermia—usually a temperature of 38°C is maintained.

Fluids

Sodium overload is a common problem in critically ill patients including burns. Following the resuscitation phase, 4% glucose/0.18% saline is used to avoid sodium overload. Although albumin may be used as a rescue solution in the acute phase, there is no convincing evidence for its use routinely.

Gastrointestinal

Wherever possible, critically ill burns patients should be enterally fed within 48 hours of admission. Such patients are at risk of stress ulceration and suitable prophylaxis with H_2 blockers should be used. Metabolic requirements for the first week are 35 mL/kg for the first week and 25 mL/kg thereafter. Bowel aperients should be given routinely to ensure regular bowel movements, which are hindered by the use of opiates and sedation.

Infection

Infection in critically ill burns patients is a major cause of morbidity and mortality, particularly burn wound sepsis and ventilator acquired pneumonia (VAP pneumonia occurring 48 hours after the onset of mechanical ventilation). These patients are at risk because of the breach in the normal protective skin barrier but also because of endotracheal tubes and intravascular catheters. Their immune system is compromised as evidenced by T-cell anergy and monocyte HLA-DR reduced expression. Close collaboration with microbiologists is essential.

Ventilator-acquired pneumonia

Various strategies have been shown to be associated with a reduction in ventilator-acquired pneumonia:
• Chlorhexidine oral gel in mechanically ventilated patients
• H_2 blockers in patients who are not fed enterally
• Use of endotracheal tubes with supraglottic suction port
• Early weaning from mechanical ventilation
• Selective decontamination of the digestive tract (SDD)

Vascular line infection

Vascular line infections are classified by the following criteria:
- Catheter-associated line infections
- Catheter-related bloodstream infections

Avoidance of vascular catheter infection is vital and helped by:
- Use of theatre cap, face mask with sterile gown, gloves when inserting indwelling vascular catheters
- Daily surveillance for possibility of line infection
- Adoption of critical care line care bundles

Metabolic

Several trials of tight glycaemic control in general critical care patients have given conflicting results in terms of improved survival, and overall there is insufficient evidence to conclude that tight glycaemic control decreases mortality. Early glycaemic control in critically ill burns patients does appear to be associated with a reduction in mortality.

Pharmacy

Input from an experienced critical care pharmacist to the care of the critically ill burns patient is vital to help with the following:
- Monitoring of drug interactions
- Monitoring of drug levels for potentially nephrotoxic drugs, eg. vancomycin
- Advice on prescribing for burns patients with drug and alcohol dependency

Renal

Acute kidney injury occurs in 25% or critically ill burns patient according to the RIFLE criteria and a third of patients with acute kidney injury will require artificial renal support (haemofiltration or haemodiafiltration for the critically ill patient). The mortality from patients with burns requiring artificial renal support is significantly increased to around 45%. Avoidance of renal failure means ensuring patients have an adequate circulating volume and adequate mean arterial pressure to perfuse kidneys; patients on antihypertensive medications often need a higher MAP.

Causes of renal failure in burns patients.

Prerenal
- Hypotension due to inadequate fluid replacement
- Hypotension from haemorrhage
- Septic shock

Intrinsic
- Rhabdomyolysis
- Interstitial damage due to nephrotoxic drugs

Post renal
- Obstruction due to blocked catheter

Further reading

Snell JA, Loh NW, Mahambrey T, Shokrollahi K. Clinical review: the critical care management of the burn patient. Critical Care 2013;17:241.

Anaesthesia: preoperative management of patients with acute burns

Introduction to anaesthesia

Aggressive fluid resuscitation and coordination of multidisciplinary care have been crucial to the dramatic improvements in survival and functional recovery of patients with major burn injuries in recent decades. The skills, knowledge base, and experience of anaesthetists match the needs of burn patients very well. Effective anaesthetic management of these patients, however, requires some understanding of unique features of pathophysiology associated with large burns. It is also important to be familiar with ICU goals for the individual patient so that perioperative interventions are compatible with the multidisciplinary care burn patients require. Close communication with the surgeons regarding the surgical plan (eg. tangential vs. fascial excision, whether open tracheostomy is anticipated, if prone positioning might be required) is necessary in order to anticipate intraoperative variables such as blood loss that are essential for decisions regarding airway management, vascular access, and monitoring.

Preoperative evaluation

Major burn injuries affect virtually every organ system. As a result, patients with these injuries present multiple challenges to the anaesthetist:
- Inhalation injury
- Difficult airway
- Altered mental status
- Limited peripheral vascular access
- Haemodynamic instability
- Rapid blood loss
- Decreased colloid osmotic pressure
- Oedema
- Altered drug response
- Impaired temperature regulation
- Infection and sepsis

In addition to the standard pre-anaesthetic evaluation, there are unique features of burn pathophysiology and surgery that require special attention because they involve increased technical challenge and/or risk.

Goals of preoperative evaluation and preparation
- Identify patients in need of immediate airway intervention and support of respiration.
- Identify fire-related systemic toxicity from inhaled substances such as carbon monoxide or cyanide.
- Determine the extent and distribution of burns, the quality of the resuscitation, presence of associated injuries, and the patient's overall physiological status in order to plan for monitoring and intraoperative management.

History

- The patient's history provides important details that will assist in planning perioperative care of patients with large burns.
- Factors that will increase resuscitation fluid requirements of burn patients:
  - Inhalation injury
  - Extensive full thickness burns
  - Delay in resuscitation (over 2 hours)
  - Electrical burns
  - Other soft tissue injuries
- Time of injury: Systemic responses to burn injuries are dynamic and pathophysiological changes vary greatly with time after injury. The haemodynamic response to burns is biphasic. Initially extravasation of intravascular fluid results in hypovolaemia, intense vasoconstriction, and decreased cardiac output. After a few days a hyperdynamic circulatory pattern develops with increased cardiac output, decreased systemic vascular resistance, and increased organ perfusion. Delays in resuscitation beyond 2 hours after burn injury increase fluid requirements for maintenance of intravascular volume as much as 50%
- Mechanism of injury: Flame burns, scalds, electrical injury, and chemical burns each involve different pathophysiological mechanisms that can require different care. Flame injuries are more likely to cause airway thermal injury and smoke inhalation, electrical injury can be associated with myocardial injury or muscle necrosis and myoglobinaemia that can lead to renal damage, and patients with corrosive chemical burns may still be contaminated with irritants that can cause injury to medical personnel if not neutralized or removed. Other unique issues can be anticipated if the mechanism of injury is known
- Risks of inhalation injury: Exposure to smoke in an enclosed space, impaired avoidance behaviour (eg. unconsciousness, extremes of age, debilitating injury, etc.), or exposure to steam or corrosive fumes are strong risk factors for inhalation injury that must be further evaluated. History of oropharyngeal scalds, especially in children, can be associated with minimal presenting symptoms but progress to airway occlusion. Patients with suspected oropharyngeal scalds should be evaluated by indirect or direct laryngoscopy or by flexible fibreoptic endoscopy for evidence of laryngeal injury and airway compromise
- Co-existing conditions: There may be additional traumatic injury in addition to cutaneous burns and inhalation injury. These injuries may require additional surgical treatment and/or may influence resuscitation. Pre-existing illness may limit the patient's physiological reserve and may alter therapeutic choices

Physical examination

- Airway: Facial burns, soot deposits, carbonaceous sputum, hoarse voice, dysphagia, drooling, respiratory distress, strider, increased effort of breathing, and other evidence of airway obstruction or respiratory failure require urgent evaluation for possible tracheal intubation and mechanical ventilation. Not all patients with inhalation injury require intubation, however, and complications of intubation include serious morbidity and death, especially during transport when unintended extubation can occur and heavy sedation or muscle relaxants may be used. In patients at risk of inhalation injury but who do not show evidence of respiratory distress or airway obstruction laryngoscopy (either direct or fibreoptic) can distinguish between patients with airway compromise who would benefit from intubation and those who do not require intubation (see Figure 5 in Muehlberger et al. Efficacy of fiberoptic laryngoscopy in the diagnosis of inhalation injuries. Archive of Otolaryngology Head and Neck Surgery 124:1003–7)
- For patients who are intubated the position of the endotracheal tube must be determined and the tube must be properly secured. Cutaneous burns and oedema of the head and neck can make it difficult to secure the endotracheal tube with confidence. In our institution nasal endotracheal tube placement is utilized and secured with one-eighth inch cotton umbilical tape looped around the nasal bony septum. This effectively secures the endotracheal tube (along with gastric and feeding tube ties) and avoids tape and circumferential ties that might irritate wounds
- Extent and distribution of injury: Extent of burn injury is expressed as % total body surface area (%TBSA) involved and is described as partial or full thickness burns (see Chapter 9 Assessment of burn surface area and Chapter 10 Burn depth assessment). Knowledge of the distribution of burns is important to anticipate difficulties with airway management, placement of vascular cannulas and monitors, and intraoperative positioning (eg. prone). Circumferential burns involving the chest may restrict chest wall motion and respiration. In this case escharotomy may be indicated to improve respiration
- Neurological: Impaired consciousness may be an indication of shock, hypoxic injury, or intoxication from inhalation of systemic toxins such as carbon monoxide or cyanide
- Extremities: Circumferential burns can restrict limb perfusion necessitating escarotomy. Burns of extremities limit access for vascular cannulation for arterial pressure monitors and intravenous fluid administration. Hypovolaemia and vasoconstriction can result in diminished peripheral pulses for 24–36 hours which can make arterial cannulation more difficult and increase risk of complications. After approximately 24 hours a hyperdynamic circulatory pattern begins to develop and peripheral pulses increase making arterial cannulation easier and safer (when indicated)

Diagnostic studies

- Chest radiograph: A chest radiograph is indicated for all burn patients at risk for inhalation injury. Although radiological findings are usually not evident soon after smoke inhalation injury, the admission radiograph is helpful as a baseline to evaluate changes as they may develop
- Blood gas analysis: For patients at risk for inhalation injury blood gas analysis with carbon monoxide oximetry can provide carboxyhaemoglobin concentration which identifies patients with carbon monoxide toxicity (levels greater than 15% toxic, more than 50% may be lethal). Acid–base status is helpful in titrating fluid resuscitation and arterial oxygen partial pressure can identify problems with pulmonary gas exchange. Persistent metabolic acidosis with apparently adequate intravascular preload may indicate carbon monoxide or cyanide toxicity
- Bronchoscopy: The diagnosis of inhalation injury is generally made on the basis of history and physical examination and confirmed with bronchoscopy findings. Oedema, mucosal damage, inflammation, bronchorrhea, and fibrinous exudates are evident with serious smoke inhalation injury. Upper airway compromise from thermal injury and/or oedema can be most effectively evaluated by endoscopy. This information is valuable for identifying patients who will benefit from early intubation or those with laryngeal injury that could be exacerbated by a translaryngeal endotracheal tube and might benefit from tracheostomy and a laryngology consultation

Quality of resuscitation

The current standard of care is early excision of burn wounds. In some centres this may be done while the initial fluid resuscitation is in progress or soon after. It is important to know if resuscitation efforts have been appropriate (avoiding over or under resuscitation) and if the patient is re-sponding favourably. There are many formulas for guiding resuscitation of burn patients (see Chapter 11 Fluid resuscitation in burns). These formulas can be used to estimate an appropriate volume of fluid the patient should receive by a given time after injury. The rates of fluid infusion estimated by these formulas are starting points and fluid administration must be titrated based on the patient's response. Intravascular volume expansion is maxi-mized when the fluid is infused over a period of time rather than as given as a bolus in a shorter interval. Some centres use an albumin solution to rescue patients who are requiring extra amounts of fluid and/or are developing oedema related complications. Quality of resuscitation can be determined from the patient's physiological status as indicated by the volume of fluid given, blood pressure, urine output, haematocrit, acid base status, and pres-ence of oedema that could be associated with compartment syndromes.

Surgical plan

Preparation for perioperative anaesthetic management must be done within the context of the surgical plan. Blood loss and problems associ-ated with patient positioning will depend on the surgical plan and these factors will influence decisions regarding vascular access, monitoring and airway management.

- Surgical technique
  - Tangential excision can be associated with bleeding that is copious and brisk
  - Fascial excision of skin and subcutaneous tissue down to muscle fascia produces less bleeding than tangential but may also be associated with extensive haemorrhage
  - Tumescent technique involves subcutaneous injection of dilute crystalloid solution with or without adrenaline to reduce bleeding and facilitate burn excision or donor site harvest; large volumes injected can add to fluid volume given and hypertension resulting from systemic effects of adrenaline may need treatment (avoid interventions that impair ventricular contractility in this case)
- Positioning: If prone positioning is required extra consideration must be given to securing the airway and vascular catheters
- Anticipated blood loss: Surgical blood loss from wound debridement and donor harvest sites increases with time after injury and with wound infection. During the first 24 hours surgical blood loss has been reported to be approximately 0.5 mL per cm^2 burn wound to be excised and grafted (where cm^2 to be excised = total body surface area × % body surface area to be excised × 10,000 cm^2/m^2). This increases over the next 2 weeks and if the wounds also become infected approximately 1.25 mL per cm^2 blood loss can be expected

Further reading

Bittner EA, Shank E, Woodson LC, Martyn JA. Acute and perioperative care of the burn-injured patient. Anesthesiology 2015;122:448–64.

Cancio LC. Initial assessment and fluid resuscitation of burn patients. Surgical Clinics of North America 2014;94:741–54.

Woodson LC, Sherwood ER, Kinsky M (eds). Anesthesia for burned patients. In Herndon DN (ed.) Total burn care, 5th edn. Edinburgh: Elsevier, 2018; pp. 131–57.

Anaesthesia: intraoperative management of patients with acute burn injury

Selection of anaesthetic agents

No specific anaesthetic technique has been found to be superior for burn patients as long as consideration is given to the expected pathophysiological changes.

Airway management

If burn injuries do not distort airway anatomy, standard induction and intubation procedures are appropriate. In the absence of sepsis, gastric emptying is not delayed in patients with severe burns. At the time of admission following injury the patient may present with a full stomach when intubation is indicated. If rapid sequence induction is necessary the question of when it is safe to use succinylcholine arises. Owing to the risk of hyperkalaemic cardiac arrest it is recommended that succinylcholine be avoided after 48 hours following burn injury until approximately 1 year after healing. This is not an absolute contraindication, however. The hyperkalaemic response to succinylcholine is highly variable and treatable. If it appears that anoxic injury due to laryngospasm is imminent, the use of a small dose of succinylcholine to relieve laryngospasm is a matter of clinical judgement.

Monitors and vascular access

Special considerations for burn patients are necessary in applying minimum standard monitors recommended by the American Society of Anaesthesiologists and decisions regarding more invasive monitors:

- Pulse oximetry: Transmission oximetry sites may be burned or within the surgical field. When available, reflectance oximetry may be used and at times pulse oximetry may be disrupted or unavailable
- Electrocardiogram: Standard gel electrodes will not adhere to burned skin or in the presence of topical antibiotic ointments. Surgical staples with alligator clips are effective in these cases
- Foley catheter: Since general anaesthesia masks most symptoms of transfusion reaction a Foley catheter is necessary if it is expected that blood products will be needed. Measurement of urine output is a common index of global perfusion. Bladder temperature is also a reliable measure of core temperature
- Venous access: Although central venous pressure (CVP) is not considered a reliable measure of cardiac preload, when replacing large volumes of blood loss in potentially septic patients it is very helpful to know if the CVP is high or low. Venous catheters should be secured with sutures and when peripheral venous access is not available central venous catheters must be large enough to allow rapid fluid flow. It is possible to place central venous catheters through burned skin but another choice is to ask the surgeon to debride the insertion site before placement
- Arterial catheter: In addition to conventional indications for placement of arterial catheters, in burn patients extremities may not be available for non-invasive cuffs because they can dislodge fresh grafts or may be in the surgical field. Radial artery catheters are difficult to maintain for extended periods in burn patients and the arms are often burned. Despite risks of femoral artery catheters this is often the preferred site when direct measurement of arterial pressure is necessary especially for prolonged periods

Fluid management

Massive crystalloid volumes administered for the acute burn injury and the addition of further crystalloid often administered with tumescent techniques during surgery, can often lead to over-resuscitation. The following methods can be utilized to reduce the volume of intraoperative fluid and blood products administered:

- Maintain spontaneous ventilation when possible. With reduced intrathoracic pressure, preload can be maintained with less volume administered. In addition, securing the endotracheal tube can be difficult in the presence of facial burns and when spontaneous ventilation is maintained, dislodgment of the tube can be corrected with less urgency
- Use of colloid solutions to replace shed blood can reduce the total fluid volume needed. Since burn patients have reduced albumin levels, 2.5 % albumin usually has the same albumin concentration as plasma. Dilution of the patient's haemoglobin with colloid solution during the initial excision reduces the red cell mass of surgically shed blood. This can reduce the amount of packed red cells needed to achieve a desired haemoglobin concentration after haemostasis is achieved
- Transfusion trigger depends on the individual patient's physiological status and co-existing diseases. With massive transfusion dilution of coagulation factors may result in coagulopathy. At our paediatric burn centre colloid solutions supplemented with packed red cells when needed are used until half the predicted total blood volume has been shed. If significant blood loss is expected to continue we then begin to replace blood loss with packed red blood cells diluted 1:1 with fresh frozen plasma
- There is no single reliable physiological endpoint to titrate fluid replacement and it is necessary to monitor several variables: systolic blood pressure, arterial pressure wave form (when arterial pressure is monitored directly), central venous pressure, urine output, haemoglobin concentration, and acid–base balance. Adequate preload must be maintained but with attention to details this can be accomplished without overload

Thermal regulation

Burn-related destruction of the major thermoregulatory organ (skin), a hypermetabolic response to large burns, and alterations in central thermoregulation including an increase in the set point (approximately 0.03°C per percent of total body surface area burned) make patients with large burns susceptible to hypothermia. This is exacerbated during surgery when the patient is completely exposed. Reduction in core temperature of burn patients, even below their elevated set point, results in a brisk hypermetabolic response. This is poorly tolerated as these patients already are experiencing an intensely catabolic stress from their wounds and the associated inflammation. The following measures should be taken to avoid hypothermia.

- Before the patient arrives the operating room should be warmed
- Overhead warmers above the patient available for use when needed
- Intravenous fluids should be warmed
- Cover areas outside the surgical field when possible
- Use 'bear huggers' or warming blankets during surgery

Postoperative care

Several issues must be addressed before postoperative care is transferred to the burn unit or surgical ICU.

Continued bleeding

Continued bleeding at donor sites and excised wounds may be significant and yet concealed by bulky dressings. This can be revealed by steady decreases in arterial and central venous pressures and changes in the arterial pressure wave form. When this is suspected, surgical advice should be sought immediately to determine if the patient requires a return to theatre to control bleeding and ICU personnel should prepare for any transfusion that may be required.

Temperature

Precautions must be taken to avoid heat loss during transport from the operating room to the burn unit. Transfer of the patient must include provisions to maintain temperature or to re-warm.

Pain

Burns are associated with intense pain. Poorly controlled pain increases anxiety, sympathetic tone, and catabolic stress. Burn pain often involves a component of neuropathic pain poorly controlled with morphine. Some patients develop rapid tolerance to morphine and experience an associated hyperalgesia. Methadone is more effective than morphine for neuropathic pain and has been found effective in burn patients tolerant to morphine and whose pain is poorly controlled by morphine. Alpha 2 adrenergic agonists (clonidine and dexmedetomidine) have also been found to facilitate analgesia in burn patients.

Further reading

Bittner EA, Shank E, Woodson LC, Martyn JA: Acute and perioperative care of the burn-injured patient. Anesthesiology 2015;122:448–64.

Cancio LC. Initial assessment and fluid resuscitation of burn patients. Surgical Clinics of North America 2014;94:741–54.

Woodson LC, Sherwood ER, Kinsky M, et al. Anesthesia for burned patients. In Herndon DH (ed.) Total burn care, 5th edn. Edinburgh: Elsevier, 2018.

Chapter 16

Burns surgery

General considerations

Following initiation of resuscitation, and the assessment of the size, depth and anatomic location of a burn injury, a plan for the ongoing treatment of the patient is formed. This may include a variety of operative strategies during the acute phase. Outlined below are those commonly used in our practice.

The benefits of operative management

Before the latter half of the twentieth century, burn wounds were managed by a prolonged period of exposure and eschar separation. This was a lengthy process, associated with multiple episodes of infection, severe metabolic disturbances, considerable pain and suffering, extended periods of hospitalization and high mortality rates. In the modern era of burns treatment, timely removal of eschar and wound closure is the mainstay of management. Better understanding of resuscitation, nutritional and respiratory support, and the management of sepsis have all contributed to improved survival rates following a large burn. Even more important was the introduction of early total excision of full-thickness burns and autograft application pioneered in the 1950s on small burns and developed throughout the 1960s and 1970s, which was associated with a dramatic decline in mortality of burns patients.[1,2]

Early excision is associated with a decreased hypermatabolic response and shorted hospital stays compared with later excision. Furthermore, as the formation of hypertrophic scars is associated with delayed healing, early excision and wound cover is indicated for any burn wound likely to take more than 10 days to heal in order to produce the best scars possible.[3] Moreover, studies have shown that early total excision does not increase the total operative time, nor the total number of blood transfusions required compared with staged excision. Rather, blood loss is less when surgery is performed within 24 hours of a major burn than it is within any point in the next 16 days.[4]

Surgical planning

Treatment planning depends on the assessment of the following factors:
• Burn size – % Total Burn Surface Area (TBSA)
• Burn depth
• Burn anatomical distribution
• Available donor site
• Patient age
• Pre-existing comorbidities and general condition of patient

Prior to starting surgical treatment of a burn, it is essential that the burns team have a clear plan of the aims and predicted sequence of operative management. The advantages gained by the early excision of major burns mean that advocates of immediate excision and grafting recommend that the maximum area possible is excised in a single operation, within the 24 hours. A more staged approach is that of early serial excision. About 25% TBSA is excised in one operation, with each stage being two days apart. The aim is to have completely excised the burn within the first five days.

Smaller burns, particularly those that are patchy or of indeterminate depth, may be delayed so that the areas that are able to re-epithelialize are allowed to do so, thus avoiding over-excising the burn. Any areas that have not healed by 10-14 days should be excised to minimise adverse scarring.

Attention is then turned to the amount of skin cover required, and the available donor sites for autograft, as well as the order of priority for each anatomical area. For smaller burns with plentiful donor site availability, the emphasis lies in minimizing donor site morbidity and maximizing cosmetic and functional outcome. Donor sites are confined to hidden areas including the thighs and scalp. Wherever possible, sheet grafts, rather than meshed grafts are used to cover burn wounds in very visible areas, such as the face and hands, to improve the cosmetic result.

In major burns where donor site is limited, the priority is covering large confluent areas as early as possible, in order to minimize the number of operative procedures and maximize survival. The sequence of areas to be autografted depends on the surgeon, with some arguing that large areas such as the posterior trunk should be covered first, and others aiming to cover functional areas such as the hands early. For all large burns the likelihood of tracheostomy requirements must be considered early, so the anterior neck can be grafted if necessary.

Areas that have been excised but not covered by autograft have allograft, biological or non-biological dressings or skin substitutes placed until such a time as autograft becomes available.

Equipment and preparation

The following requirements should be considered, and equipment made available before surgery is carried out on a burns patient.

General requirements

As a rough guide for patients with larger burns, it is expected that one operation will be performed for every 10% TBSA burn wound. This is only achieved with a clear plan from the outset, with an established order of priority and plan. An experienced surgical team, consisting of surgeons, anaesthetists, and scrub nurses enables the smooth progression of the operation, minimizing theatre time, and the detrimental effect to the patient.

Temperature

The environmental temperature of the operating room should be maintained at around 30°C, which can be achieved by ambient heating as well as radiant heaters over the operating table. Fluids for washing should be warmed, and areas not being operated on should remain covered. This limits hypothermia and its sequelae, including detrimental effects to coagulation. Regular measurements of the patient's temperature throughout the procedure must be performed, and surgery stopped if hypothermia persists to allow for a period of rewarming.

Infiltration

Pre-debridement tumescence with 1:1,000,000 epinephrine solution under burn eschar is useful for limiting bleeding in areas where a tourniquet cannot be used. Similar infusion subcutaneously to proposed donor sites reduces blood loss and aids donor site harvest.

Blood products and minimizing blood loss

Significant blood loss is inevitable in all large burn operations, and must be anticipated for.[5] Cross-matched packed red cells should be available before starting surgery. The use of pneumatic tourniquets during excision of burns to limbs, topical phenylephrine soaks applied following excision, and the wrapping and elevating of limbs all reduce blood loss. Permissive hypotention and administration of fresh frozen plasma, or recombinant factor VIIa may also be used.

Skin preparation

Once the patient is anaesthetized, all dressings are removed. Due care must be taken to minimise heat loss during this time. The patient is washed with a warm aqueous povidone–iodine solution and lose eschar or tissue removed, before being rinsed with warm water. Soiled drapes and dressings are removed before povidone–iodine surgical preparation is applied and fresh sterile drapes placed. For major burns, the whole body is washed in this way, at the start of the operation. This is aided by dividing the team initially into a "dirty" and "clean" scrub team.

Knives

A variety of knives may be required for excision. Scalpels are required for sharp debridement. Horizontally mounted skin graft knives for shaving skin include the Watson modification of the Humby knife for larger areas and the Goulian knife for small and tricky areas. These should be to hand, alongside the necessary blades required for each. Most skin graft knives have adjustable apertures to set the desired depth, whereas the Goulian has a series of blade guards that are changed according to the depth of excision required.

Water jet systems

The Versajet® consists of a single use hand piece connected to a high pressure pump system and a foot pedal. This generates a stream of saline parallel to the wound surface, creating a Venturi effect. This cutting effect debrides the wound surface by creating a local vacuum while simultaneously aspirating debris back into the handpiece.[6]

Dermatomes

Skin grafts may be harvested using the skin graft knives described above. However, for larger areas, it can be difficult to obtain grafts of consistent depth using these instruments. An electric or air-driven dermatome helps the burn surgeon to harvest split thickness skin grafts of uniform thickness. The thickness of the graft can be set by adjusting the aperture of the dermatome. Typical depth is set at 10/1000 inch, but thicker or thinner grafts may be required depending on the donor site and area to be grafted. Guards between 2 and 4 inches wide may be fitted to set the width of the graft.

Cadaveric skin and skin substitutes

Careful planning is required to anticipate the need for expensive products such as cryo-preserved skin and skin substitutes (discussed below). It is useful to calculate the surface area that will be required before beginning excision so the necessary amounts can be located, and prepared. Cryopreserved skin must be defrosted and cannot be reused.

Meshers

Meshers create multiple fenestrations throughout sheets of graft, allowing expansion of the graft and enabling the cover of large areas of wound. Furthermore, the holes created allow blood or seroma beneath the graft to escape. There are broadly two types of mesher: those producing a fixed mesh ratio and those that use dermacarriers on boards to produce the mesh ratio. The ratio (1.5:1, 2:1, 4:1, etc.) implies the amount of expansion that may be achieved, although in practice this is usually less than expected.

Fixing grafts

Following the application of a graft to a wound, it must be secured. This may be achieved using sutures, which are typically absorbable, or staples. In general absorbable sutures are used for cosmetically sensitive areas, such as the face. Staples are extremely useful, particularly for larger burns, as they limit the operative time significantly. Tissue glue and topical surgical sealants such as Tisseel may also be used.

Burn excision

The chosen technique to excise a burn depends on the depth of the burn. In partial thickness burns, the aim is to preserve as much viable dermis as possible, in order to improve the appearance and suppleness of the resultant scar. In full thickness burns, where no dermis remains, speed and the production of a viable bed that will readily accept a graft are of paramount importance.

Tangenital excision

Described by Janzekovic in 1975, this technique allows the excision of the superficial, devitalized layers of burn eschar, while preserving the healthy deeper dermis beneath.[7,8] A skin graft knife or dermatome is used to sequentially shave layers of deep partial thickness burn until viable tissue is reached. This is manifest by the appearance of punctate dermal bleeding. The finer and more numerous the bleeding vessels in the resultant wound bed, the more superficial the burn. Thrombosed vessels or a purple appearance indicate further excision is needed to achieve a graftable bed. These appearances are particularly useful when a tourniquet is being used and bleeding is not evident.

Full thickness excision

A Watson knife or dermatome is used to excise the full thickness of the skin in one pass, to the underlying fat. Viable fat is seen as yellow and glistening, in contrast with red fat containing thrombosed vessels. Alternatively, a scalpel or monopolar diathermy may be used to sharply excise non-viable skin. This is particularly useful when contour preservation is important, such as on the face, or when the maintenance of underlying structures is desired.

Fascial excision

An alternative for burns extending through all or most of the fat or in large infected wounds is the excision of the full thickness of skin and subcutaneous fat, onto fascia. This fascial plane is relatively avascular, rendering an added benefit of greatly reduced blood loss. Furthermore, fascia is an excellent bed for grafting, and will readily accept skin grafts. Unfortunately, this method of excision is very mutilating, with total loss of contour and the excision of all lymphatic channels. This produces poor cosmetic results and lymphoedema in the long term.

Hydroexcision

Hydroexcision using a water jet surgical tool (the Versajet®) is a useful alternative to standard excision of mid to deep dermal burns using knives. It creates a smooth wound bed, which is particularly useful on areas that are difficult to excise such as the face and hands. It has the added advantages of maximizing dermal preservation by accurately removing devitalized tissue while preserving healthy tissue, especially useful for mixed depth burns. It simultaneously removes necrotic and infective debris, thus creating a clean bed to receive grafts or biological dressings. For this reason it is commonly used for debridement of granulating wounds or prior to application of Biobrane®.

Amputation

Very deep burn injuries, often due to high voltage electrical current, may lead to significant muscle involvement. The resultant necrosis and rhabdomyolysis can be life threatening. While every attempt at limb preservation is made, amputation is sometimes necessary in the presence of renal failure or an ischaemic limb or digit.

Enzymic debridement

Enzymes of plant (such as bromelain from pineapples) or bacterial origin have been studied for their potential to selectively debride necrotic burn eschar while preserving healthy tissue and minimizing bleeding. The results have proved to be highly variable.

Wound closure

Following burn wound excision, the closure of the resultant wound must be addressed. This reduces pain, evaporative water loss, infection, heat loss and promotes healing. Autograft is a permanent method of wound closure, but when donor sites are scarce, temporary methods may be used until such a time as donor sites have regenerated enough to be reharvested.

Autograft

These may be either full thickness or split thickness skin grafts. Full thickness grafts are confined to relatively small burns as the donor site requires direct closure, although harvesting larger areas by using cosmetic techniques such as abdominoplasty has been described. However, full thickness skin grafts require optimal wound conditions to ensure take: not usually possible following an acute burn. Full thickness grafts are extremely useful for post-burn reconstruction.

Split thickness skin grafts are much more commonly used for immediate wound cover. These are harvested with either a skin graft knife or dermatome. They may be used as sheet graft or meshed, and applied with absorbable sutures or staples.

Allograft

Allograft is harvested from cadaveric donors following routine screening for communicable disease. To maintain viable cells it may be stored either refrigerated in nutrient medium for a week, or frozen in a cryoprotectant medium containing glycerol. This method preserves 85% viability of cells after a year. Alternatively, non-viable allograft is produced by preserving it with higher concentrations of glycerol or freeze-drying. Rarely, allograft is harvested from living donors immediately prior to its use.

Allograft may either be used as a sheet graft on cosmetic areas such as the face, or meshed 2:1, but not expanded, to prevent desiccation of the underlying excised wound. Alternatively it is over 4:1 meshed autograft when donor site is severely limited creating a 'sandwich graft', protecting the underlying autograft as re-epithelialization occurs.[9]

Biological dressings

Biological dressings may be organic or synthetic. Organic dressings include skin harvested from other species (xenografts), usually porcine, and human amnion. The synthetic biological dressing Biobrane® is a bilayer consisting of an outer silicone sheet and an inner nylon mesh impregnated with porcine collagen. It decreases pain of partial thickness burns while promoting re-epithelialization. It can also be useful following debridement of full thickness burns until a donor site is available, or for donor sites. Biobrane® is however extremely susceptible to infection. It must therefore be used within 24 hours of injury, applied following meticulous debridement and cleaning, and antibiotic cover given. It should be closely monitored for signs of infection and removed if necessary.[10]

Skin substitutes

An ongoing area of research and innovation is the creation of semi-biological and synthetic skin substitutes that allow temporary wound closure while affording further advantages such as promoting healing and or providing reconstitution of part of the skin.[11]

Integra® is a matrix containing bovine collagen and shark cartilage glycosaminoglycan. It is permanently incorporated into the wound bed. It may either be applied as a single layer, or a bilayer, with an overlying silicone membrane to reduce water vapour loss while providing temporary cover. It is usually applied acutely as a bilayer following excision of full thickness burn. The presence of infection prevents the adherence of the Integra®, and it should be inspected daily for purulent collections beneath its surface. Over 3 weeks, the matrix is vascularized and appears peach coloured. At this time, the silicone layer is removed and very thin autografts are applied to the 'neodermis', creating permanent wound closure. If successful, the scar is more pliable and less hypertrophic than that achieved by using split skin graft alone.[12]

Alloderm® is de-epidermalized de-cellularized sterile human dermis that also provides a dermal replacement. It is applied at the time of excision and wound bed preparation and a thin skin graft is applied over it. Matriderm® is a matrix of bovine dermal collagen and elastin, also placed beneath autograft in a single-stage procedure. Again, these techniques are susceptible to the presence of infection these products are more commonly used in the burns reconstruction setting.

Cultured autologous cells

Epidermal keratinocytes may be cultured in over 3–4 weeks, enabling a 1 cm^2 biopsy sample to cover a 1 m^2 area.[13] The resultant graft is however, very fragile, and even following graft take blisters easily. In order to overcome these problems, attempts have been made to graft the cultured epithelial autograft (CEA) onto an allograft dermal bed. In general the use of CEA is limited to patients with massive burns >90% TBSA where donor site is extremely limited.

More recently, ReCell®, a rapid autologous cell harvesting and processing system has been developed. This processes a skin biopsy over approximately 30 minutes, which is then sprayed onto burn wounds and donor sites.[14] It has been shown to accelerate healing and improve pigmentation of the resultant scar.

Skin grafts

As the gold standard of burn wound cover, the process of take and maturation of split thickness autografts must be understood.

Graft take

A graft is defined by being devitalized and requiring revascularization from
its recipient bed. Skin grafts go through a sequence of adherence, imbibi-
tion, inosculation, and, later, remodelling.

On application to a viable bed, fibrin bonds rapidly form, creating adherence. In the first 2–4 days following application, the graft swells as fluid is
absorbed or imbibed, into the graft by osmosis. This may contribute to the
nutrition and viability of the graft, and is more successful the thinner the
graft. Over the following 3–4 days, vessels from the wound bed anastomose
with those within the graft. This may be via inosculation (direct anastomosis
between the vessels in the bed and those in the graft); revascularization
(new vessel ingrowth from the bed along the vascular channels of the graft);
or neovascularization (new vessel ingrowth from the bed along new channels in the graft).

Adherence and take depend on the viability of the recipient bed, with
freshly excised or fresh granulating wounds accepting grafts more readily
than chronic granulation or contaminated wounds.

Graft maturation

Following graft take, a number of stages are passed before the graft ma-
tures. Initial scaling and desquamation renders grafts dry and requiring
frequent moisturization until the function of the sweat and sebaceous
glands return to a varying degree. Thicker split skin or full thickness grafts
will transfer hair to the recipient site, and this must be considered when
selecting a donor site. Re-innervation of grafts is also variable.

Problems with grafts include hypertrophic scarring and contraction.
Hypertrophic scars form around the edges of grafts, and in the interstices
of mesh grafts. Contraction is inversely proportional to the amount of
dermis available, either in the wound bed following tangential excision, or
in the skin graft itself. Some of the newer dermal substitutes aim to address
this issue. Sustained contraction around joints or anatomical landmarks may
lead to contractures, whereby functional or cosmetic deformities require
correction. A further problem with skin grafts is variable pigmentation
of both the donor and recipient sites, which can become either hypo- or
hyperpigmented.

Techniques to improve take

Seroma or haematoma formation between the graft and the recipient bed
prevents adherence of the graft. Meshing skin grafts allows fluid to escape
from beneath the graft, but may produce hypertrophic scars between the
interstices. For this reason sheet grafting is used on areas such as the face
and hands. As a compromise, the addition of small holes or fenestrations
allows some seroma or haematoma escape. Alternatively, suturing the graft
to the underlying recipient bed at multiple sites, or 'quilting' the graft, may

also prevent fluid accumulation beneath the graft. It is also useful in securing the graft in areas such as the face that are difficult to dress.

Shear forces may also disturb fibrin bonds, or the anastomotic connections between the graft and the bed. These can be prevented by the use of dressings such as tie-over bolsters to secure grafts to difficult or mobile areas. They may consist of gauze, proflavine soaked wool, or sterile foam sponge sutures to the surrounding skin. Dressings to limbs include paraffin-impregnated gauze, covered with layers of gauze dressing and crepe bandages. Over the trunk, an elasticated net dressing may be used. If necessary, splints are used to immobilise joints near to grafts to prevent movement and maintain a safe position during graft take.

Usually grafts are inspected on day 5 post grafting, with sedation if the area is extensive. Staples can be removed at this time. Good take is indicated by a pink adherent graft, with evidence of epithelialization between the interstices of meshed graft. If there are concerns about infection or haematoma, early graft checks can be carefully performed on day two. Purulent exudate may be removed and topical antimicrobials applied.

Donor sites

Donor sites are essentially superficial partial thickness injuries and heal by epithelialization from the remaining epithelial appendages such as hair follicles and sweat glands in seven to 10 days. The thicker the graft harvested, the slower the healing, with a higher hypertrophic scar formation.

Guide for specific burns

Burns of different sizes and depths and in different anatomical areas are all managed using a variety of the above techniques. Each patient must be managed on an individual basis, but examples of strategies for surgical management following commencement of resuscitation and stabilization are provided.

Small to medium superficial partial thickness burns

Superficial partial thickness burns <40% TBSA, presenting within 24 hours of injury are often managed using Biobrane®. Under sedation or anaesthesia, cleaning and debridement of burned epithelium is performed, followed by application of Biobrane® and dressings which are removed at 24 hours for inspection. If the Biobrane® is adherent at this time, no further dressings are required. As re-epithelialization occurs in 10–14 days, the Biobrane® spontaneously separates from the wound and is trimmed.

Alternatively, topical Silvadene (1% silver sulfadiazine), biological dressings, conventional dressings such as paraffin impregnated gauze or silicone sheet, or other synthetic dressings are applied and changed regularly until the wound heals.

Large superficial partial thickness burns

Burns >40% are more prone to contamination and infection and can have a high morbidity despite their superficial nature. For this reason, allograft is often used to achieve temporary cover following debridement. Once the patient is stabilized, this is replaced in a staged manner by autograft. Alternatives to allograft are the use of other biological dressings as described above.

Deep partial thickness burns

Whether large or small, early total wound excision and grafting is the preferred method of treatment for deep burns in order to limit the inflammatory response. Where possible, the dermis is preserved by the use of tangential excision, and the wounds are covered with autologous split skin grafts. If donor sites are limited, temporary wound closure is achieved with allograft, biological or semi-biological dressings until the donor site heals sufficiently to re-harvest.

Alternatives are serial excision of the amount of burn wound that can be closed by the available donor site. Unexcised areas are treated with topical antimicrobials until the donor site becomes available. In particular, Flammacerium (silver sulfadiazine and cerium nitrate) can be useful as it creates a hard impermeable eschar, which decreases fluid loss, invasive wound infection, morbidity and mortality. This may be useful in patients who are unfit for total surgical excision in the initial stages.[15]

Full thickness burns

Again, regardless of size, prompt total excision and wound closure of full thickness burns reduces morbidity and mortality. Burns <10% TBSA, or larger burns that present early may be amenable to tangential or sharp excision preserving fat. However, patients with burns through some or all of the fat, or those with colonized or infected wound may require fascial excision to obtain a graftable bed. Fascial excision also limits blood loss in massive burns. The timing of excision of very large burns is imperative, as blood loss in the first 24 hours post burn is up to half of that when surgery is performed after this time. However, performing total excision of a burn >40% TBSA is undeniably a huge undertaking requiring numerous surgeons, anaesthetists and nurses. Units without these resources may choose to excise in several staged operations.

As before, autograft, meshed as necessary, is the preferred wound cover. For larger burns 'sandwich grafts' may be necessary. Alternatively, allograft or the biological or semi-biological dressings discussed above may be used as temporary wound cover, or permanent dermal replacement. These wounds are subsequently covered with autograft as it becomes available.

Anatomical areas of special consideration

The face and neck are areas of cosmetic and functional importance. Even deep burns of the face are usually treated with topical antimicrobials or repeated allograft application until a viable wound bed is apparent. Very rarely are burns excised, in order to preserve as much contour and viable tissue as possible. Medium to thick split skin sheet autografts are used in aesthetic units, with quilting sutures used to preserve anatomical landmarks.

The glabrous skin of the hands is thick, highly specialized and usually heals. It is thus best to manage burns to the palm relatively conservatively. The dorsal skin is thin and usually requires excision and sheet grafting. Initially the hands should be splinted in a position of safety. Following graft inspection at 5 days, gentle mobilization can commence.

Meshed split skin grafts should be placed onto the trunk with the interstices running horizontally. In the limbs, the meshed interstices should run longitudinally. The exception to this is around joints, where they should be perpendicular to the axis of the limb and not expanded.

References

1. Barrow RE, Herndon DN. History of treatment of burns. In Herndon DN (ed.). Total burn care. Philadelphia, PA: Saunders Elsevier, 2007; pp. 5–6.
2. Herndon DN, Barrow RE, Rutan RL, et al. A comparison of conservative versus early excision therapies in severely burned patients. Annals of Surgery 1986;204:547–53.
3. Deitch EA, Wheelahan TM, Rose MP, et al. Hypertrophic burn scars: analysis of variables. Journal of Trauma 1983;23:895–8.
4. Desai MH, Herndon D, Broemeling L, et al. Early burn wound excision significantly reduces blood loss. Annals of Surgery 1990;221:73–762.
5. Hart DW, Wolf SE, Baeuford RB, et al. Determinants of blood loss during primary burn excision. Surgery 2001;130:396–402.
6. Klein MB, Hunter S, Heimbach DM, et al. The Versajet water dissector: a new tool for tangiental excision. Journal of Burn Care & Rehabilitation 2005; 26:483–87.
7. Janzekovic Z. A new concept in the early excision and immediate grafting of burns. Journal of Trauma 1970;10:1103–8.
8. Muller M, Gahankari D, Herndon DN. Operative wound management. In Herndon DN (ed.) Total burn care. Philadelphia, PA: Saunders Elsevier, 2007; pp. 179–80.
9. Alexander JW, MacMillan BG, Law E, et al. Treatment of severe burns with widely meshed skin autograft and widely meshed akin allograft overlay. Journal of Trauma 1981;1:75–78.
10. Baret JP, Dziewulski P, Ramzy PI, et al. Biobrane versus 1% sulver sulfadiazine in second-degree paediatric burns. Plastic and Reconstructive Surgery 2000;105:62–5.
11. Jeschke MG, Finnerty CC, Shahrokhi S, et al. Wound coverage technologies in burn care: novel techniques. Journal of Burn Care & Research 2013;34:612–20.
12. Heimbach DM, Warden GD, Luterman A, et al. Integra dermal regeneration template for burn treatment. Journal of Burn Care & Rehabilitation 2003;24:42–8.
13. Munster MA. Cultured skin for massive burns. A prospective, controlled trial. Annals of Surgery 1996;224:372–5.
14. Gravante G, Di Fede MC, Araco A, et al. A randomized trial comparing ReCell system of epidermal cells delivery versus classic skin grafts for the treatment of deep partial thickness burns. Burns 2007;33: 966–72.
15. Garner JP, Heppell PS. The use of Flammacerium in British burns units. Burns 2005;31:379–82.

Burn wound dressings

Goals of burn healing

The ultimate goal for all burns is to allow the wound to heal with the least amount of scarring, and this is directly related to the depth of burn injury. Superficial partial thickness burns and deeper burns of small area can be treated by suitable dressings alone and this is probably the most widely applied form of treatment for burns. Superficial partial thickness burns will heal by re-epithelialization from the keratinocyte reserve within the epidermal appendages, while smaller deeper burns will heal by a combination of wound contraction and re-epithelialization from the wound edge. In both cases, this can be supported and promoted by wound dressings, after appropriate debridement and cleansing. Numerous studies have shown that re-epithelialization occurs more rapidly in a moist wound environment and if there is no barrier to this cell migration such as clot, slough or infection.

Definitive vs. temporary dressings

Initial cover of the burns wound after initial first aid needs to be simple, widely available, and effective to maintain the wound in a clean state, reduce pain, and protect from the external environment. Cling film is widely regarded as the best option in the first instance, although most marketed simple dressings such as Tulle gauze (Jelonet) and similar are reasonable options. Dressing ointments such as Flamazine should be avoided in the initial phase if transfer to a burns unit is required as it alters the appearance of the burn and making it difficult to assess.

The ideal definitive burn dressing

There are many characteristics of the ideal wound dressing (Box 17.1) and these principles can be applied to burn dressings. The key features of dressings that are required by burns surgeons include lack of adhesion, ease of pain-free dressing change, absorbency, and antimicrobial activity. Currently there is a lack of evidence to guide clinicians as to the 'gold-standard' dressing for burn injury.

Box 17.1 Characteristics of the "ideal" wound dressing

[1] Maintain a moist environment at the wound–dressing interface
[2] Absorb excess exudate without leakage to the surface of the dressing
[3] Provide thermal insulation
[4] Provide mechanical and bacterial protection
[5] Allow gaseous and fluid exchange
[6] Absorbent to wound odour
[7] Non-adherent to the wound and easily removed without trauma
[8] Non-toxic, hypoallergenic and non-sensitizing to the patient and medical professional
[9] Sterile
[10] Cost-effective and easily available

Dressing composition

In essence, all dressings consist of three components. There is a non-adherent interface layer that lies in direct contact with the wound surface, and this can allow wound interaction by the addition of compounds such as antimicrobials or biomolecules. Next, there is an absorbent layer that can sequester wound exudate and store it away from the wound interface, providing the essential 'moist' wound environment rather than a 'wet' wound. Finally, there is an adhesive layer that will allow the fixation of the dressing to the patient, and importantly, not to the wound, regardless of burns size or anatomy. Such dressings may be prefabricated by a manufacturer, and some such dressings may combine all of these properties into a single layer dressing (eg. the hydrocolloids) which have variable adhesion depending upon wound moisture levels and inbuilt absorbency. While pre-fabricated, or composite, dressings are a useful 'off the shelf' commodity, the variety of dressings that are available worldwide allows a specific tailor-made dressing to be created on a patient-by-patient basis. The combination of different interface layers, with topical antimicrobials; a variable degree of absorbency, which will depend upon wound exudate; and specific adhesive properties, depending upon the size of the burn wound and the anatomy involved, as well as such issues as hypersensitivity to specific dressings allows dressings to be varied according to wound microbiology, as well as clinician and patient requirements.

Interface layer

Non-adherent dressings

Typically a fine meshed material, either dry or combined with a hydrophobic agent. This will include the polyethylenes (eg. Telfa clear®), silicones (eg. Mepitel®) and impregnated gauze (eg. Jelonet®). These can all be combined with topical antimicrobials.

Silver

Silver has a long history as an antimicrobial agent dating back to antiquity. Since the 1970s, silver has been delivered in the nitrate from, or in combination with a sulphonamide antibiotic. More recently, the development of nanocrystalline silver, consisting of both silver oxides and metallic ions, has allowed enhanced solubility and controlled release of silver giving a broad spectrum of activity against Gram-positive and Gram-negative species, as well as yeasts and fungi. Silver sulfadiazine (synthesized from silver nitrate and sodium sulfadiazine) is the most commonly used prophylactic agent in burns dressings and is manufactured as a 1% concentration in a water-soluble cream base (Flamazine®). Local hypersensitivity has been reported, as well as transient leukopenia at 3–5 days post burn. Cerium nitrate silver sulfadiazine (Flammacerium®) is indicated for larger deep burns in patients who may not be candidates for early surgical debridement. The cerium appears to be beneficial because of its effect on the eschar rather than wound infection, producing a tougher eschar that may seal the wound more effectively than silver sulfadiazine. Nanocrystalline silver dressings (eg. Acticoat®) consist of a flexible rayon/polyester sheet bonded to a polyethylene mesh and coated with a film of silver which will elute over time when exposed to wound exudate, allowing dressings to be left in place for longer. Silver-containing dressings may exhibit toxicity to keratinocytes and fibroblasts. Currently, there is insufficient evidence to establish whether silver-containing dressings or topical agents promote wound healing or prevent wound infection.

Iodine

Although iodine has a broad spectrum of activity of action against Gram-positive and Gram-negative species, as well as yeasts and fungi, it has been shown to have potential toxicity to fibroblasts and keratinocytes and is rarely used in routine burn wound dressings. It may be applied as povidone-iodine solution (eg. Betadine®) or in combination with a knitted viscose fabric (Inadine®).

Other

Mupirocin (Bactroban®) has a spectrum of action against MRSA and poly-myxin B/bacitracin (Polyfax®) in combination have activity against Gram-positive and Gram-negative species, and are commonly used for superficial burns to the face as well as infected wounds. Honey can improve healing times in superficial and partial thickness burns compared with some conventional dressings.

Biosynthetics

Biobrane® is a bilaminate dressing, comprising a silicone membrane bonded to a layer of nylon fabric mesh and coated with a monomolecular layer of type 1 collagen of porcine origin. It is designed to adhere to the wound until re-epithelialization is complete, providing flexible semi-occlusive membrane through which the wound can be observed. It is indicated for superficial partial thickness burns (eg. scalds), especially in the paediatric age group, and can be manufactured as anatomical garments. It is also useful in desquamating skin conditions such as toxic epidermal necrolysis.

Absorbent layer

Absorbent gauze can be tailored to the level of wound exudate, but will need changing when saturated. A hydrogel is a network of polymer chains that are hydrophilic and highly absorbent. Their ability to absorb more than their own weight in fluid allows provision of a moist wound environment, preferential to wound healing. Hydrogels include the alginates (Sorbsan®, Kaltostat®) and synthetic carboxymethylcellulose (Aquacel®, Intrasite®), which can incorporate silver (eg. Aquacel®Ag).

Adhesive layer

The adhesive layer will secure the dressing in place, reducing shearing forces, thus providing comfort, reducing evaporative heat losses and acting as a protective barrier to the injured tissues. These include the occlusive polyurethane film dressings (Tegaderm®, Opsite®), and the semi-occlusive polyester tapes (Mefix®, Hypafix®), employing acrylic adhesives. Dressings can also be secured in place with sutures or surgical staples for areas that are prone to shearing or dressing dislodgement.

Negative Pressure Wound Therapy

Negative pressure wound therapy (NPWT) is the application of a negative pressure across a wound to aid wound via drainage of excess exudate and increasing localized blood flow. It is a three-component dressing consisting of an interface layer, absorbent layer (which is drained by negative pressure) and an occlusive film (VAC®, Renasys®). Currently, there is a lack of evidence about whether NPWT therapy is effective in the treatment of partial thickness burns.

Summary of burn wound dressings

Burns that are selected for treatment by dressings alone, or in combination with surgical debridement and skin grafting, require regular monitoring, both clinically and microbiologically. Wound photography allows a record to be made of wound progression. Modern dressings may allow a longer interval between dressing changes, but this should not be sacrificed in favour of regular review. If wound healing progresses at the expected rate, then the comfort afforded by fewer changes of dressings is advantageous, but the poorly progressing wound should be treated aggressively with a custom-designed dressing which can be tailored for the individual needs of the patient.

Further reading

Greenhalgh DG. Topical antimicrobial agents for burn wounds. Clinics in Plastic Surgery 2009;36:597–606.

Selig HF, Lumenta DB, Giretzlehner M, et al. The properties of an "ideal" burn wound dressing – what do we need in daily clinical practice? Results of a worldwide online survey among burn care specialists. Burns 2012 38:960–6.

Wasiak J, Cleland H, Campbell F. Dressings for superficial and partial thickness burns. Cochrane Database of Systematic Reviews 2008;4:CD002106.

Management of burn wound infection

Introduction

Changes in the management of burn wounds popularized by Herndon. brought a paradigm shift in the typical infecting aetiology and progression of disease. Associations to development of Gram-negative burn wound infection include increased total body surface area (TBSA), Abbreviated Burn Severity Index (ABSI), Acute Physiology And Chronic Health Evaluation, version 2 (APACHE-2) scores, and length of hospital stay. The presence of multiple such factors warrants a high index of suspicion and should be included in risk assessment. Human resource planning, including designation of clinical microbiology, infection control, and specialized cleaning/housekeeping staff in day-to-day management of burn patients is crucial. Meticulous attention to hand hygiene continues to be imperative in reducing cross-contamination rates, however, evidence regarding 'bare below the elbow' policies is scant and contended.

- Early wound excision, skin grafting, and shower therapy are the mainstay of modern burn care and result in significantly reduced infection rates
- Pre-1990 mainstays of treatments such as delayed burn excision, immersion hydrotherapy, and eschar separation have been largely abandoned
- These techniques remain in practice in a minority of burn centres, and are associated with significantly increased rates of burn wound infection

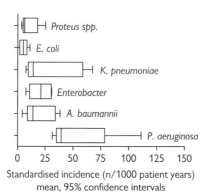

Standardised incidence (n/1000 patient years)
mean, 95% confidence intervals

Fig 18.1 Standardized incidence of Gram-negative pathogens infecting burn wounds in civilian adult hospitalized patients

Bacterial dynamics and trends in burn wound infection

The choice of appropriate antibiotic therapy during the turn-around time until definite results of microbial culture and sensitivities are received has a significant bearing on outcome of the infection itself as well as wound healing. It is therefore appropriate to consider the changes in natural microbial burn wound dynamics over time and specific factors which suggest an increased index of suspicion for particular pathogens. Particular considerations in initiating antibiotic therapy include

- Gram-positive pathogens predominate the early post-burn infection period (Figure 18.1)
- Streptococcal spp., even ≤10 CFU/mL may cause total graft loss
- Gram-negative infection predominates after the fifth post-burn day
- *Pseudomonas aeruginosa, Acinetobacter baumannii, Escherichia coli, Enterobacter* spp., and *Proteus* spp. are associated with the majority of Gram-negative infection
- Tetanus status, vaccination, and administration of human tetanus immune globulin should be ascertained on admission
- Anaerobe cover is recommended, especially in patients with concurrent blast injury

A series of pathogens is associated with particular patterns of injury, increased antimicrobial resistance, and fulminant deterioration.

- Post-burn contact with untreated water, typically to extinguish flames, is a principal risk factor for *Aeromonas hydrophila*. Other associations with *A. hydrophila* reported in the literature include younger, adult, males with TBSA >40%, and full thickness burns
- *A. hydrophila* is an obligate symbiont of *Hirudo medicinalis*, which is finding increased favour in plastic surgery units to treat venous congestion post tissue transfer
- Aeromonas is largely resistant to co-amoxiclav and treatment with quaternary fluoroquinolones is recommended as the treatment of choice
- *Cedecia lapigei* tolerates high pH and classically occurs in association with chemical injury arising from slaked lime (calcium hydroxide), a component of several types of mortar, cement, and render in the construction industry
- *Stenotrophomonas maltophilia* infection is another opportunistic emerging pathogen associated with burn injury. Although uncommon, rapid (within hours) deterioration has been associated with this organism, and signs of infection classically include refractory leukaemoid reactions, thrombocytopenia, acute renal, myocardial failure, and endotoxic shock

Management

Gram-staining is a cost-effective, rapid, and well-established technique that provides essential information to guide initial antimicrobial chemotherapy until the microbial culture and sensitivity results are available. Microscopic examination may determine the infecting species by morphologic examination. Common sensitivities to guide initial antimicrobial therapy are reported in Table 18.1. The availability of a clear, concise local antimicrobial policy, where available, is essential to fine-tune general principles of management to local resistance patterns, as is round the clock access to clinical microbiology and diagnostics.

Table 18.1 Common antimicrobial agents used for treatment of burn wound infection

Pathogen	Common first-line antimicrobial chemotherapy*
Gram-negative pathogens	
Pseudomonas aeruginosa	Fluoroquinolones (eg. ciprofloxacin)
Acinetobacter baumannii	Carbapenems (eg. imipenem)
Escherichia coli	Cephalosporins eg. cefotaxime
Klebsiella pneumoniae	Carbapenems (eg. imipenem)
Enterobacter spp.	Aminoglycosides (eg. gentamicin)
Proteus spp.	Cephalosporins (eg. cefotaxime)
Aeromonas spp.	Fluoroquinolones (eg. ciprofloxacin)
Stenotrophomonas maltophilia	Co-trimoxazole, polymyxin
Gram-positive pathogens	
Staphylococcus (MSSA)	Penicillins, cephalosporins, macrolides
Staphylococcus (MRSA)	Glycopeptides (eg. teicoplanin)
Streptococcus spp.	Penicillins

*Where present, local antimicrobial chemotherapy sensitivities and guidelines should be considered

Last-line therapy and recent innovations

Colistimethate sodium (colistin) is a venerable antibiotic whose fortunes have been revived with the rise of multidrug-resistant bacteria. Low resistance rates continue to be reported. However, increased resistance has been observed with *Klebsiella* spp. and pseudomonas spp. in the Asia-Pacific, Latin American, and central European regions.

- It acts in a detergent fashion on bacterial cell walls, is bactericidal, and reports excellent activity against multidrug-resistant bacteria, with rapid reduction in absolute bacterial counts
- However, this effect is brief and in vitro rapid regrowth has been observed even at 2–6 hours post dose. This needs to be borne in mind considering the wide variation of dosing intervals in the literature
- Expert support is warranted given widely varying manufacturer recommended doses:
  - 2.5–5 mg/kg (31,250–62,500 IU/kg) per day, divided in two to four equal doses (USA)
  - 4–6 mg/kg per day, divided into three doses for adults and children (>60 kg), and 80–160 mg/8 hours if <60 kg (UK)
- Various dosing intervals are reported in the literature from 4–36 hours, and doses vary up to 720 mg/day parenterally divided in three doses/24 hours
- Bacterial recovery occurs early following administration of colistin, suggesting that increasing the frequency rather than the dose may be beneficial in decreasing the viable bacterial load
- "On-the-shelf" hydrolysis of colistin methanesulfonate (CMS) is an underestimated and easily preventable aspect of CMS toxicity, with fatalities being reported in the literature. Therefore, CMS administration should be performed promptly on reconstitution
- Side effects include nephrotoxicity and neurotoxicity
- Synergistic action with other drugs such as rifampicin has been reported

Given its extensive spectrum against Gram-negative bacteria and exquisite sensitivity, intensive research efforts have been directed at altering the activity/toxicity balance of the colistin molecule. Azzopardi et al. have recently reported that chemically coupling colistin to large dextrin polymers successfully reduced toxicity while allowing size-based passive targeting towards the infected site. Most of colistin's toxicity relates to its extensive positive charge, and novel colistin derivatives bearing reduced positive charges have also shown promise in recent trials.

Multiple co-existent injury, such as blast injury, amputation, and degloving injury, warrants a consideration of anaerobic, gas-forming organisms. Tetanus immunity should be determined on admission and human tetanus immune globulin administered as per Emergency Management of Severe Burns guidelines (EMSB) or their local equivalent.

Fungal and viral infection

Several factors in burn injury contribute to an immunosuppressed state, and consequent emergence of opportunistic viral and fungal infection. Concurrent multiple trauma, malnutrition due to gastroparesis, and inhalational injury compliment the well-established immunosuppressive effect of major burns (>30% TBSA). This provides fertile grounds for growth of opportunistic organisms including fungi and viruses.

Fungi are ubiquitous and together with the host immunosuppression, caused by the thermal injury, may lead to fungal wound infections (FWIs).

- Fungi encountered in burn infections include, Mucormycosis, Aspergillus, Fusarium, and Trichosporonosis
- 20–25% of burns wound infections are caused by fungi. Burns are colonized with both yeasts and fungi, especially Candida although the latter rarely invade the wound. The invasion usually occurs from the second week onwards

Since burns may lead to immunosuppression one may experience clinically significant viral infections in such cases. The viruses implicated usually belong to the Herpes group of viruses and include Herpes simplex virus (HSV), Cytomegalovirus (CMV), and Varicella zoster virus (VZV).

- HSV typically presents with a vesicular rash which appears along the base or the margins of the wound. This usually appears after the first week of burn infections. These lesions then rupture and ulcerate with or without forming a crust
- HSV predominantly infects burns in the nasolabial area and usually affects healing partial thickness burns. Recommended treatment in such cases is aciclovir, eg. 5 mg/kg IV for 7–10 days
- Prophylactic use of aciclovir in facial burns is not yet a documented recommendation although its use is recommended for facial resurfaces
- Human cytomegalovirus is known to infect full thickness burns due to its opportunistic potential. The infection may occur in both seropositive and in seronegative patients either due to primary infection or due to reactivation
- Allograft skin may be infected with CMV
- Commonly recommended treatments for fungal infections are illustrated in Table 18.2

Table 18.2 Treatment options for fungal infections

Mucormycosis	First line: amphothericin B (liposomal) 5–10 mg/kg/day Amphotericin B 1–1.5 mg/kg/day Second line: posaconazole 400 mg po BD with meals
Aspergillus	Variconazole 6 mg/kg/day BD day 1 then 4 mg/kg/day BD IV
Fusarium	First line: amphothericin B (liposomal) 5–10 mg/kg/day Amphotericin B 1–1.5 mg/kg/day Second line: posaconazole 400 mg po BD with meals

*Local clinical microbiology guidelines and advice should be consulted

Topical antibacterial therapy

Wound dressing with topical antimicrobial agents may provide an effective adjunct in the management of infection.

- Silver-based topical antimicrobials such as silver sulfadiazine act principally via competitive inhibition of bacterial or fungal dihydropteroate synthesis
- These bacteriostatic agents offer both Gram-positive and Gram-negative coverage by preventing folic acid synthesis, inhibiting growth
- Topical antimicrobials are absorbed systemically, to some degree
- Silver sulfadiazine is contraindicated in patients suffering from glucose-6 phosphatase deficiency (G6PD)
- White cell counts should be monitored for transient leucopenia
- Silver topical therapy may also slow down wound healing
- With the exception of mafenide acetate, topical antimicrobials work best after excision, as eschar penetration is poor
- Other topical antimicrobials in use are summarized in Table 18.3. Candidates in development are listed in Table 18.4.

Table 18.3 Topical antimicrobial agents used in management of burn wound infection

Topical antimicrobial	Target	Notes
Silver sulfadiazine	Broad spectrum (Gram-positive, Gram-negative, fungi)	Poor eschar penetration Caution in G6PD; Monitor WCC (see text) Can damage cornea. Bacteriostatic/bactericidal
Cerium nitrate (commonly with silver as Flammacerium®)	Antimicrobial contribution of cerium nitrate is contended	Cerium nitrate binds to and then denatures lipid protein complexes, preventing immunosuppression
Silver nitrate 0.5%	*Staphylococcus* and *Pseudomonas* spp.	Monitor Na+ and K+ hyponatraemia and hypokalaemia have been reported
Nanocrystalline silver (several formulations)	Reduces wound infection and promotes wound healing	Metastable, high energy form of silver which is more soluble in solution. This higher solubility may result in different properties such as reduced toxicity and improved antibiotic activity
Nystatin (fungistatic)	Antifungal (fungistatic), binds to cell membrane sterols, increasing permeability	Poor systemic absorbtion; excreted unchanged in faeces
Sodium hypochlorite (Dakin's solution)	Broad spectrum 0.025% solution is bactericidal	Germicidal antiseptic wetting agent; dissolves necrotic tissue debris; May impair wound healing at higher concentrations agents like dakin's solution and mafenide acetate might not be widely available in some countries

Table 18.3 (Contd.)

Topical antimicrobial	Target	Notes
Mafenide acetate 10%	Gram-positive bacteria	Deep tissue penetration, significant systemic absorbtion. Carbonic anhydrase inhibitor: tends to precipitate hyperchloremic metabolic acidosis. Monitor ABG, avoid if TBSA >20%
Acetic acid (aqueous) solution	*Pseudomonas aerugionsa*	Caution in large burns, monitor pH due to risk to acetate toxicity and metabolic acidosis
Povidone iodine	Iodine is active against a wide variety of bacteria, fungi, protozoa, and viruses	Mix of molecular iodine and polyvinylpyrrolidone. Iodine present in the complex is the active agent
Cadexomer iodine		Hydrophilic starch powder containing iodine, which is a suitable dressing for granulating wounds such as venous ulcers
Liposomal iodine		Purported advantage of microbicidal activity of iodine with the tolerability liposomes
Enzyme alginogels	Bacteria/fungi/ yeasts	Contain enzymes glucose oxidase, lactoperoxidase providing antimicrobial activity.

Some agents, like sodium hypochlorate may not be readily available in some countries.

Table 18.4 Topical agents in development

Agent		Notes
Chitosan	Hydrogel	Polycationic polymer of glucosamine which acts in a detergent fashion on bacterial memtbeanes to cause destabilization.
	Film	
	Bandage	Chitosan rapidly clots blood. FDA approval as haemostatic agent attained
Antimicrobial peptide	Defending Scorpion B	Antimicrobial peptides also act via an amphiphilic structure with a polycationic hydrophilic moiety as well as a hydrophobic moiety
	Demegel rBPI	
	Histone Ceragenin	
Miscellaneous	Superoxidized water	Based on hypochlorous acid
	BCTP nanoemulsion	An oil-in-water nanoemulsion. Composed of polyoxyethylene-sorbitan monolaurate or polyoxyethyl-enesorbitan monooleate (surfactant) with 8% ethanol, 64% oil, 1% cetylpyridinium chloride and distilled water
	Acidified nitrite	Releases nitric oxide and other reactive nitrogen intermediates
Bacterophage therapy		Limited by specificity to species and strain of bacteria

Dosing regimens: specific considerations in major burns

Significant fluid shifts may be caused by major burns, especially within the first 24 hours post burn, especially third-space fluid accumulation and due to variations in total body water, intracellular and extracellular volume, plasma volume and its constitution. Thermal injury has the potential to result in hypovolaemia and haemochromaturia, which entail an impairment of renal function. Hypoalbumenaemia may rapidly set in despite gastrointestinal support affecting total protein binding. These factors must be borne in mind when considering the effective volume of distribution of administered antibiotics, their bound/unbound fractions, and effective concentrations at the infected site.

Conclusion

This chapter provides an overarching view of best-evidence management and care for infected burn patients. Burn infection is still the major cause of morbidity and mortality in burn patients. Appropriate attention may substantially reduce the impact of infection on the overall stability of the burn patient and specific aspects of wound healing. The importance of clinical microbiology input into the burn multidisciplinary team is paramount.

Further Reading

Azzopardi EA, Azzopardi E, Camilleri L, et al. Gram negative wound infection in hospitalised adult burn patients-systematic review and metanalysis. PloS one 2014;9:e95042.

Azzopardi EA, Azzopardi SM, Boyce DE, Dickson WA. Emerging Gram-negative infections in burn wounds. Journal of Burn Care & Research 2011;32:570–6.

Azzopardi EA, Boyce DE, Thomas DW, Dickson WA. Colistin in burn intensive care: Back to the future? Burns 2013;39:7–15.

Azzopardi E, Ferguson E, Thomas D. A novel class of bioreponsive nanomedicines for localised re-instatement of bioactivity and specific targeting. The Lancet 2014;383:S9.

Azzopardi EA, Ferguson EL, Thomas DW. Colistin past and future, a bibliographic analysis. Journal of Critical Care 2012;28:219.

Azzopardi EA, Ferguson EL, Thomas DW. The enhanced permeability retention effect: a new paradigm for drug targeting in infection. Journal of Antimicrobial Chemotherapy 2013;68,257–74.

Azzopardi EA, Whitaker IS, Rozen WM, et al. Chemical and mechanical alternatives to leech therapy: a systematic review and critical appraisal. Journal of Reconstructive Microsurgery 2011;27:481–6.

Bond L, Clamp P, Gray K, Van Dam V. Patients' perceptions of doctors' clothing: should we really be 'bare below the elbow'? Journal of Laryngology & Otology 2010;124:963–6.

Bazaz R, Brown C. War on white coats. Lancet 2007;370:2097.

Capoor MR, Sarabahi S, Tiwari VK, Narayanan RP. Fungal infections in burns: diagnosis and management. Indian Journal of Plastic Surgery 2010;43:S37.

Church D, Elsayed S, Reid O, et al. Burn wound infections. Clinical Microbiology Reviews 2006;19:403–34.

Fong J, Wood F. Nanocrystalline silver dressings in wound management: a review. International Journal of Nanomedicine 2006;1:441.

Gales AC, Jones RN, Sader HS. Contemporary activity of colistin and polymyxin B against a worldwide collection of Gram-negative pathogens: results from the SENTRY Antimicrobial Surveillance Program (2006-09). Journal of Antimicrobial Chemotherapy 2011;66:2070–4.

Garner J, Heppell, P. Cerium nitrate in the management of burns. Burns 2005;31:539–47.

Herndon DN. Total burn care, 3rd edn. New York: Elsevier, 1996.

Leung C, Drew P, Azzopardi EA. Extended multidrug-resistant Stenotrophomonas maltophilia septicemia in a severely burnt patient. Journal of Burn Care & Research 2010;31:966.

Ozkurt Z, Ertek M, Erol S, et al. The risk factors for acquisition of imipenem-resistant Pseudomonas aeruginosa in the burn unit. Burns 2005;31:870–3.

Rabea EI, Badawy ME-T, Stevens CV, et al. Chitosan as antimicrobial agent: applications and mode of action. Biomacromolecules 2003;4:1457–65.

Richardson MD, Warnock DW. Fungal infection: diagnosis and management. Chichester: Wiley, 2012.

Schlag S, Nerz C, Birkenstock TA, et al. Inhibition of staphylococcal biofilm formation by nitrite. Journal of Bacteriology 2007;189:7911–19.

Shoji H. Extracorporeal endotoxin removal for the treatment of sepsis: endotoxin adsorption cartridge (Toraymyxin). Therapeutic Apheresis and Dialysis 2003;7:108–14.

Vaara M, Sader HS, Rhomberg PR, Jones RN, and Vaara T. Antimicrobial activity of the novel polymyxin derivative NAB739 tested against Gram-negative pathogens. Journal of Antimicrobial Chemotherapy 2012;68(3):636–639.

Wasiak J, Cleland H, Campbell F. Dressings for superficial and partial thickness burns. Cochrane Database of Systematic Reviews 2008;4:CD002106. doi: 10.1002/14651858.CD002106.pub3.

Whitaker IS, Kamya C, Azzopardi EA. et al. Preventing infective complications following leech therapy: is practice keeping pace with current research? Microsurgery 2009;29:619–25.

Whitaker IS, Josty IC, Hawkins S, et al. Medicinal leeches and the microsurgeon: a four-year study, clinical series and risk benefit review. Microsurgery 2011;31:281–7.

Wibbenmeyer L, Danks R, Faucher L, et al. Prospective analysis of nosocomial infection rates, antibiotic use, and patterns of resistance in a burn population. Journal of Burn Care & Research 2006;27:152–60.

Wong TH, Tan BH, Ling ML, Song C. Multi-resistant Acinetobacter baumannii on a burns unit—clinical risk factors and prognosis. Burns 2002;28:349–57.

Chapter 19

Chemical burns

Introduction to chemical burns

Chemicals cause 2.4–10.7% of all burn injuries worldwide; burns from chemicals are seven times more common in males than females. Although relatively rare, these injuries account for up to 30% of burn deaths, and therefore demand careful and timely management. Recent studies suggest that improved health and safety measures may be reducing the incidence of industrial injuries but domestic injuries are increasing. Head and neck structures, including eyes, and extremities are most commonly affected. The most important step in the intial management of a chemical burn is the immediate removal to halt further injury. Thereafter, the management is similar to other burn injuries although some chemicals require specific management steps, discussed below.

Classification

Chemicals which cause burns can be grouped into six main classes according to their mechanism of action. These are summarized in Table 19.1.

However, the most important clinical distinction is between acidic and alkalotic burns. Acids (pH 1–7) donate protons (H^+) in solution and alkalis (pH 8–14) accept hydroxyl ions (OH^-). Examples of strong acids (pH < 2) include sulphuric acid (H_2SO_4) and hydrochloric acid (HCl), which are both corrosive and also a desiccant and a reductant respectively. Injurious alkalis usually have a pH > 11.5 and include cement. The remaining causes of chemical burns can be largely classed as organic or inorganic solutions.

Table 19.1 Classes of burning chemicals according to mechanism of action

	Mechanism of action	Examples
Reductants	Electron donors	HCl, nitric acid, alkyl mercuric compounds
Oxidants	Accepts electrons	Sodium hypochlorite, potassium permanganate, chromic acid
Corrosives	Denature proteins on contact	Phenols, cresols, lyes, H_2SO_4, HCl, sodium metals
Protoplasmic poisons	Form esters with proteins or bind/inhibit vital organic ions such as calcium	Ester formers: formic and acetic acid, inhibitors: oxalic, hydrofluoric acid
Desiccants	Dehydrate tissues	H_2SO_4 and concentrated HCl
Vesicants	Ischaemia leading to anoxic necrosis; forms blisters	Mustard gas, DMSO, Lewisite, cantharides

DMSO; dimethylsulfoxide

Pathophysiology

Chemicals denature proteins by disrupting the weak bonds that maintain the protein's tertiary three-dimensional structure. Acids, apart from hydrofluoric acid, cause coagulation necrosis upon contact with skin, resulting in the formation of an eschar or coagulum. This limits the amount of acid that penetrates underlying tissue. However, alkalis usually produce more severe wounds as they cause liquefaction necrosis of cutaneous tissue, allowing alkalis to react with underlying fat and other tissues. Alkalis tend to manifest the true extent of injury days after initial insult. Therefore, thorough examination and evaluation for involvement of deeper tissues is warranted in cases of alkaline chemical injury. Organic solutions dissolve lipid cell membranes and thereby disrupt cell architecture while inorganic solutions damage skin by direct binding to injurious agents and salt formation with proteins.

Clinical features

The severity of the resulting burn injury is dictated by the substance responsible, its phase (air, liquid, or gas), quantity and concentration, duration of exposure and total body surface area (TBSA) burnt, subsequent management, regional skin properties and mechanism of action. A thorough history and physical examination may reveal some of these factors and are therefore warranted. A high index of suspicion for concealed injury should also be maintained.

Clinical features can be general to all chemical burns or specific to particular substances or classes of substances.

General features

Skin and appendages
Mottled dry or wet skin; may develop blisters; partial and/or full thickness burn

Gastrointestinal
Oral burns or oedema; drooling; abdominal pain; guarding; dysphagia: there is an increased likelihood of perforation and oesophageal strictures.

Ophthalmic
Decreased visual acuity; diplopia; corneal abrasion; corneal opacification: this increases risk of blindness.

Respiratory
Respiratory arrest; stridor; wheezing; dyspnoea; tachypnoea; use of accessory muscles; subcutaneous air (Haman's crunch).

Workup

Investigations

Full blood count; urea and electrolytes; liver function tests; blood urea nitrogen; serum creatinine; coagulation profile; urinalysis: myoglobinuria; arterial blood gas (ABG) analysis; electrocardiogram; also see Table 19.1 for specific investigations depending on the chemical involved. Suspicion of ocular injury mandates fluorescein and slit-lamp examinations.

Imaging

Chest X-ray if respiratory symptoms; abdominal X-ray: supine and erect if suspected peritonitis.

General management principles

The principles of managing chemical burns are generally similar to thermal burns, but special considerations are to be made regarding initial management of chemical burns.

Removal of chemical from skin

- Remove particulate debris, brush off dry chemicals, and remove all potentially contaminated clothing. Carers should wear protective clothing to avoid injury.

Hydrotherapy with appropriate drainage

Copious irrigation with water for duration of at least 30 minutes to 2 hours may be required. Immersion into a tub is not recommended as chemical containment exacerbates burn injury. Examine for signs of hypothermia; maintain room temperature between 28°C and 31°C and lavage water near body temperature. Caution is advised on relation to neutralizing the chemical as this may induce a biochemical reaction, thereby precipitating further injury, but specific neutralizing agents for chemical injuries do exist and are widely available especially in industry, such as Diphoterine. Diphoterine is of particular value as it is effective against a range of chemical classes, including acids and alkalis, and can be used on th skin, eyes and has been used for esophageal burns.

Correct estimation of the extent of injury

- Depth and TBSA of burn.

Identification of systemic toxicity

- Acid/base imbalances should be identified early. Hydrofluoric acid in particular can cause systemic derangement including hypocalcaemia and resultant ventricular arrythmias such as Torsades de Pointes and ventricular fibrillation. Other biochemical derangements such as hypomagnesia and hyperkalaemia can also occur and compound the risk of death even with HF burns of <1% TBSA.

Treatment of ocular contacts

- Copious irrigation is required and an ophthalmologic consult should be made. Fluorescein staining to assess corneal or scleral abrasions. Assess pH of the eyes. Diphoterine may also be used to irrigate eyes. pH may also be used to assess adequacy of irrigation: aim for pH 7.0–7.3.

Management of chemical inhalation injury

- Acute airway inflammation and necrosis may occur after caustic ingestion. Consider establishing a definitive airway if the patients is in respiratory distress. All chemical inhalation burns should be reviewed early by an Anaesthetist.

Special considerations for specific agents

Assaults using corrosive substances

- Often referred to as 'acid attacks' although attacks may be from caustic (alkali) or acids.

- Recent published guidelines describe the three Rs: remove (clothing), rinse (copiously with water), and report (to emergency services).
- After first aid management, care should be delivered at specialist burns services.

Table 19.2 Specific features and management

Substance (industrial uses)	Features/workup	Special management points
Chromic acid (laboratory glassware cleaning, chromium plating)	Non-painful corrosive ulcers; may cause respiratory distress if inhaled; monitor for systemic effects as even 10% TBSA burns are often fatal; blood urea nitrogen; creatinine	Irrigation ± phosphate buffer solution in an industrial setting. For systemic effects, dimercaprol 4 mg/kg IM for 2 days then 2–4 mg/kg/day for 7 days. Dialysis lowers chromium blood levels
Hydrofluoric acid (glass etching, oil refinery)	Damage may appear minimal initially; can cause cardiorespiratory, neurological and gastrointestinal effects. Subungal tissues are particularly prone. Monitor Ca^{2+}, K^+, Mg^{2+} and ECG (long Q-T syndrome)	Treatment is in four stages: hydrotherapy with water (or hexafluorine lavage); topical treatment (eg. Ca^{2+} gel); infiltration of 0.5 mL of 10% calcium gluconate per cm^2 and radial arterial infusion of 10 mL of 10% calcium gluconate and 40 mL 5% dextrose solution over 2–4 hours, until cessation of pain
Phosphorous (water treatment plants, pesticides)	ECG: cardiac arrhythmias; Ca^{2+}; PO_4^-	White phosphorous ignites with oxygen; identify and remove phosphorous particles using phosphorescence or 0.5% $CuSO_4$, which turns particles black; important to keep the wound moist, eg. with a water-soaked gauze dressing or petroleum jelly
Oxalic acid (dyes, bleaches)	Limits muscle contraction; monitor urea and electrolytes, calcium ion levels; cardiopulmonary function monitoring	Irrigation and IV Ca^{2+}
Nitric acid (fertilizers)	Yellow-brown staining of skin and formation of a coagulum	Irrigation then topical silver sulphadiazine. Gauze dressings or occlusive, antiseptic moist bandages are used to maintain wound moisture depending on burn depth

Subsequent care

The subsequent management of chemical burns follows similar principles to management of other burn types. Begin initial assessment and management using trauma resuscitation protocols such as ATLS or EMSB. Depending on the extent of the burn, fluid resuscitation and pain management protocols are as described (electrical injuries chapter). Urine output is one of the key markers of adequate resuscitation. Once the patient is stabilized, early excision and grafting are indicated to improve outcomes if deep dermal or full thickness burns are sustained. Psychological input may be required at an early stage.

Complications

Scarring, poor wound healing, local infections, cataract formation, loss of vision.

Further reading

Palao R, Monge I, Ruiz M, et al. Chemical burns: pathophysiology and treatment. Burns 2010;36:295–304.

Tan A, Bharj AK, Nizamoglu M, et al. Assaults from corrosive substances and medico legal considerations in a large regional burn centre in the United Kingdom: calls for increased vigilance and enforced legislation. Scars, Burns & Healing 2015;1:2059513115612945.

Electrical injuries

Introduction to electrical injuries

Electrical injuries account for 3–5% of all admissions to major burn centres. Injuries often involve deeper tissues in addition to skin, resulting in high morbidity and mortality.

Classification

- Low voltage (<1,000 volts)—primary involvement of skin and surrounding tissue
- High voltage (>1,000 volts)—associated with underlying deep tissue injury including muscles, nerves, tendons, and bone
- Lightening injury—contains millions of volts of electricity lasting 1/10th to 1/1000th of a second. The pathognomonic sign of a lightning strike is a dendritic, arborescent, or fern-like branching erythematous pattern on the skin (Lichtenberg figures)

Electricity is categorized into alternating current (AC) and direct current (DC). AC is considered more dangerous as it causes muscle tetany. Flexor muscles are generally stronger than extensors, forcing the subject to hold on to the source of current rendering them unable to let go. Alternatively, DC contact results in a singular rigorous muscle contraction, often thrusting the victim away from the source.

Pathophysiology

The three major mechanisms of electricity-induced injury are as follows:
- Electrical energy causes direct tissue damage and alters cell membrane resting potential
- Electrical energy is converted into thermal energy, causing permanent tissue destruction and coagulative necrosis
- Mechanical injury with direct trauma resulting from falls or violent muscle contraction

Electrical burns may cause injury via direct contact, electrical arcs, flame, or flash injury.

Severity of injury is inversely proportional to the cross-sectional area of the body part involved. Thus the most severe injuries are often seen at the wrist and ankle with severity decreasing proximally.

Clinical features of high voltage injuries

When performing the physical examination, remember to keep a high index of suspicion for concealed injury.

Integumentary

'Kissing burn' at the flexor creases; Lichtenberg figures in lightening injury; mouth burn (age <4).

Neurological

Transient confusion; amnesia; paraesthesia; seizures; paralysis; autonomic dysfunction.

Cardiovascular

Arrhythmias: DC current usually causes asystole while AC current usually causes ventricular fibrillation; arrest; direct cardiac damage.

Respiratory

Respiratory arrest: due to either chest wall muscle paralysis or injury to the respiratory control centre in the brain.

Musculoskeletal

Compartment syndrome; avulsion fractures; costochondritis; rhabdomyolysis.

Renal

Acute kidney injury.

Workup

Investigation and treatment of electrical injuries depends on whether a high-voltage or low-voltage injury has been sustained. When it is not clear, assume a high-voltage injury and full workup.

Investigations

Full blood count; electrolytes; liver function tests; blood urea nitrogen and creatinine; urinalysis: urine myoglobin; creatinine kinase; serum myoglobin; arterial blood gas (ABGs); cardiac enzymes; ECG: The most common abnormalities seen on ECG are sinus tachycardia, non-specific ST- and T-wave changes, heart blocks, and prolongation of the QT interval. Indications for cardiac monitoring include (a) loss of consciousness (b) ECG abnormality and/or evidence of ischaemia, (c) documented dysarrythmia either before or after admission to the ED, (d) CPR at the scene of injury.

Imaging studies

Patients who are found unconscious require cervical spine, chest, and pelvis X-rays. X-rays of the extremities may be required when injury is apparent. Head, neck, chest, abdominal, and pelvic computed tomography scans may be required in individual cases.

Compartment syndrome

A low threshold for decompression is required in suspected cases. Clinical features include pain with passive motion (non-localized, severe, deep, exaggerated), paraesthesias, pallor, paralysis, and poikilothermia. Loss of pulse is a late finding. Examinations for the aforementioned signs/symptoms should commence immediately after injury and again with regular intervals within the first 48 hours post burn as this time frame has the highest risk for the development of increased compartment pressures.

If suspected, fasciotomy is immediately warranted.

Immediate care

It is of utmost importance to establish safety at the scene of injury before providing care. As with all trauma injuries, begin the initial assessment with primary survey of airway, breathing, and circulation.

Fluid resuscitation

Fluid resuscitation should commence as soon as possible. Hourly assessment of urinary output is mandatory. If urine is tea coloured or dark, myoglobinuria is likely. These patients should be aggressively resuscitated with Hartmann's solution to maintain urine output of approximately 100 mL/h or greater in an adult to minimize tubular obstruction. Mannitol is administered for osmotic diuresis. Sodium bicarbonate can be used for the alkalinzation of urine. If myoglobinuria is unlikely, resuscitation with Hartmann's solution to produce a urine output of >0.5 mL/kg/h is appropriate. Urine myoglobin levels are monitored.

   Cardiac injury is assessed by ECG, troponin levels, and echocardiography. Muscle injury is assessed by creatinine phosphokinase and myoglobin levels. Skeletal injury is assessed by physical examination and X-rays. Neurological injury is assessed by examination and head CT.

Inpatient care

Admission to a specialized burn unit is warranted in all high voltage and lightning injuries. Admission following low-voltage electrical injury is selective.

Wound care

Wound care of an electrical injury is similar to care for burn injury. Silver sulfadiazine is used as a topical agent.

Fasciotomy

Fasciotomy of the injured area is required in suspected cases of compartment syndrome as it serves as both a diagnostic and therapeutic tool. A second examination is performed 24–48 hours later. The decision to debride the wound or amputate is made at this time. If debridement is chosen, all devitalized and necrotic tissue is removed. Indeterminate tissue is left for re-evaluation 1–2 days later.

Complications

Infections, persistent arrhythmias, compartment syndrome, cataracts, acute kidney injury, complex regional pain syndromes, neurological injury, neuropathic pain, rhabdomyolysis, need for amputation.

Further reading

Arnoldo BD, Purdue GF. The diagnosis and management of electrical injuries. Hand Clinics 2009;25:469–79.

Rai J, Jeschke MG, Barrow RE, Herndon DN. Electrical injuries: a 30-year review. Journal of Trauma 1999;46:93–6.

Radiation burns

Introduction to radiation burns

Radiation burns are caused by ionizing radiation, as electromagnetic radiation (X-rays or gamma rays) or particles (alpha or beta) measured in grays (Gy). Ionization produces free radicals, causing DNA damage, cell death, and malignant change.

Radiation burns may be a consequence of radiotherapy or medical imaging using beam energy. Although rare, they can be caused by intentional radiation release such as a nuclear weapon, additionally causing eye or thermal injuries and should be included in the total body surface area (TBSA); they can also result from accidents, such as the Fukishima nuclear reactor disaster, Japan 2011. Burns from isotopes (^{192}Iridium or ^{60}Cobolt) used for brachytherapy are more common.

Radiation is emitted evenly from a source. The amount of radiation encountered decreases rapidly with distance (intensity α 1/distance^2). As radiation passes through matter, eg. tissue, it transfers energy to it (linear energy transfer (LET)). The higher the LET, the higher the absorbed radiation dose, measured in grays, with increased ionization of biological tissue (Table 21.1).

Table 21.1 Radiation types

Particle	Penetration	Skin effect
Alpha α	Little penetration. Travels a few cm in air and stopped by clothes or a sheet of paper Very high ionization	Unable to penetrate horny skin. Harmful if inhaled, ingested or prolonged skin contact
Beta γ	Higher range. Travels less than a metre in air and can be stopped by a 1-cm sheet of aluminium	Localized but severe skin damage
Gamma γ	Poor ionization. High penetrance, travelling far distances, requiring centimetres of lead or metres of concrete	Dependent on power of γ ray
Neutron	High kinetic energy, ready penetrance	Often lethal with high cell damage causing unsalvageable skin damage and necrosis
X-ray	Longer wave length than γ	Dependent on power of X-ray

Data sourced from Waghmare CW. Radiation burn – From mechanism to management. Burns 39(2):212–19, Copyright © 2013 Elsevier Ltd and ISBI, with permission from Elsevier

Localized irradiation

Signs of skin damage are progressive and dependent on total exposure. Assessment of severity is difficult due to delayed signs requiring frequent review. Medical radiation therapy is fractionated with the maximum dose focused a minimum of 0.5 cm below the surface to spare normal tissue. Higher doses (>25 Gy) are absorbed by the skin, causing collagen deposition and radiation fibrosis.

First-degree thermal burn equivalent

- >2 Gy: Mild transient erythema with onset in minutes to hours, resolving in 48 hours, eg. in sustained interventional radiology procedures >2 hours
- >6 Gy: Recurrence of more severe erythema after 2–3 weeks with dry desquamation or hair loss. Larger doses affect sebaceous glands causing dry scaly skin

Second-degree thermal burn equivalent

- >18 Gy: Moist desquamation of the skin with blisters after a few weeks. This may resolve up to 50 days after exposure or develop into necrosis

Full-thickness burn

- >25 Gy: Initially pruritus and rash, full-thickness skin ulceration and skin necrosis may occur from vascular insufficiency as cumulative exposure irrevocably damages the microvascular structure. May encompass underlying structures such as muscle

Whole-body irradiation

Acute radiation syndrome
- 1–4 Gy: Describes the whole-body effect of radiation, beginning within hours of exposure with fatigue, fever, headache, nausea, vomiting, and diarrhoea. A latent period (up to 3–5 days) follows this with other overlapping syndromes. Time from exposure to symptom onset can help estimate clinically the patient's total radiation dose

Haematopoietic syndrome
- Exposure 1–4 Gy: Bone marrow is sensitive to radiation, resulting in pancytopaenia, with haemorrhage (thrombocytopenia) and opportunistic infections (granulocytopaenia)

Gastrointestinal syndrome
- 1–12 Gy: Onset of watery diarrhoea within hours as gut epithelium is damaged, allowing bacterial translocation and sepsis, bowel ischaemia and third spacing of fluids causing hypovolaemia and acute renal failure

Neurovascular syndrome
- 15–30 Gy: Irradiation causes profound hypovolaemia from inflammatory mediators and nitrous oxide release or loss of vascular epithelium. Variable neurological symptoms are noted, with cardiovascular collapse, respiratory distress and death.
- Bone marrow failure may occur at exposure of 30 Gys and a radiation dose of 40 Gy is inevitably fatal

Immediate management

- The immediate intervention should be to prevent further patient exposure and skin ionization. In a major incident, swift triaging is required. Usually, a major radiation exposure that is survivable is not immediately lethal and concomitant injuries should be prioritized according to ATLS guidelines
- Healthcare workers should limit their time near the source and wear personal protective equipment (PPE). Radioactive material is very unlikely to be a risk to emergency or medical personnel
- Casualties must be removed from the area of greatest radiation contamination to limit exposure, if possible upwind and in the open air. Typically, casualties with suspected radiation exposure would receive decontamination near the scene, unless requiring immediate hospital treatment. Most contamination will be confined in outer clothing, which should be removed where possible, from head to foot, to minimize inhalation risk. Underwear should also be removed if suspected of contamination
- Wounds should be irrigated with plentiful amounts of saline to dilute radioactive particles. Abrasive decontamination should be avoided if possible. Care should be given not to spread contaminated fluid to unexposed tissue and showers are more appropriate than bathing the patient. Irrigation should be continued until minimal readings or no further change is found with a Geiger counter
- Patients should be treated under strict isolation precautions. Health care workers treating or assessing such patients should have all skin covered, wearing full gowns, with a mask, cap, shoe covers, and double gloves, changing in an anteroom. Outer gloves should be changed frequently, to avoid spreading contaminants to the patient's normal tissue and to avoid cross-contamination. Discarded protective gear and contaminated items should be removed after use and placed in clearly marked plastic containers for disposal. Geiger counters or other radiation detection devices should be used to assess treatment areas regularly to detect contaminants requiring decontamination
- On assessment, a full blood count should be taken immediately and at 12 hours post exposure. A lymphocyte reduction by more than half or lymphopaenia indicates a significant radiation exposure, with the patient at risk of opportunistic infections. A patient's radiation exposure can be estimated by the onset and severity of clinical symptoms along with the concentration of dicentric chromosome aberrations in peripheral lymphocytes

Further treatment

Owing to vascular damage and reduced basal cell density (>20 Gy) radiation wounds are often non-healing and susceptible to infection and sepsis.

• Anti-emetics effective in radiotherapy such as ondansetron may be useful in radiation nausea
• Radiation burns should be kept clean with washing and well hydrated to prevent further desquamation. Exposure to chemical or physical irritants or sunlight should be avoided
• Steroid (beclomethasone spray) or hydrophilic (alovera) creams significantly reduce moist desquamation, with equal effectiveness
• Moist desquamation should be treated as a burn wound, swabbed and covered
• Radiation burn wounds may be difficult to close surgically with grafting due to poor microvasculature and low capillary density. Conservative treatment should be used initially, treating other sequelae of radiation exposure. Other definitive management options including free flaps may be necessary
• Marrow failure will likely require bone marrow transplantation

Further reading

American College of Surgeons. Advanced trauma life support (ATLS) course manual. Chicago: ACS.
Waghmare CW. Radiation burn – from mechanism to management. Burns 2013;39.212–19.
Waselenko, MacVittie TJ, Blakely WF. Medical management of the acute radiation syndrome: re-commendations of the Strategic National Stockpile Radiation Working Group. Annals of Internal Medicine 2004;140:1037–51.

Chapter 22

Ocular burns

Clinical findings in ocular burns

Burns to the orbit are an inevitable consequence of the exposure of the eyelid, conjunctiva, cornea, and internal orbit to external physical and chemical irritants. Accidental exposure to dangerous chemicals can take place at the workplace or at home, with commonly used products such as detergents and cleaning agents containing acids or alkalis. Children and adults are both at risk of accidental and non-accidental orbital burns.

Although it is important to ascertain the circumstances under which an orbital burn was sustained, a focused history and examination can be commenced while simultaneously administering first aid. The prognosis of an orbital burn is dictated by the time and concentration of chemical contact with the orbit and the initial early decontamination regime performed.

Key steps in first aid

- Provide immediate early orbital lavage with water, ampohteric or neutralizing solutions
- Take protective measures such as gloves
- Open the eye with the help of an assistant or the patient if they are motivated
- Initiate lavage using a flushing technique before commencing drop-by-drop applications every second for at least 15 minutes
- Examine the deep fornices while rinsing the lids and conjunctiva Encourage the patient to carry out eye movements to all extreme positions
- Remove any visualized foreign bodies using a soft cotton swab.
- Carry out orbital lavage for 15 minutes ensuring precise time keeping
- Apply antibiotic gentamycin and steroidal dexamethasone eye drops following lavage
- Refer to Ophthalmology

Disadvantages of delayed first aid

- Continued damage secondary to burn
- Significantly poorer visual prognosis
- Increased incidence of corneal opacity, non-healing ulcers, and glaucoma

First aid

Rinsing solutions

Features

- Important for decontamination of corrosives
- A polyvalent solution is needed for effective decontamination as contents of the spill may be unknown
- Many different solutions are available on the market

Amphoteres

Features

- Chemically reactive towards acids and alkali
- Act within the frame of known biochemical activity like amino acids.
- Special solutions are available on the market distributed by Prevor Int.
- Diphoterine® has a proven high decontamination capacity of alkali, acids, alkylants, solvents, tear gas, capscain, oxidants, and reductors

Water

Features

- Freely available
- Polyvalent but not buffering
- Dilution of spills due to hypo-osmolar nature of water creating a concentration gradient
- Dilution is effective when used early in exposure to reduce concentration levels within the tissue

Buffers

Features

- Many buffers available on market
- Borate buffer more effective in akalis
- Phosphate buffer more effective in acids
- Special highly concentrated phosphate buffers are available as 'pH neutral' to deal with acids and alkalis alike
- Complication of phosphate buffer use in orbital burns includes secondary corneal calcification and is therefore not recommended

Anti-hydrofluoric acid therapies

Features

- Hydrofluoric acid acts on calcium and magnesium levels causing severe tissue necrosis and arrhythmias
- Decontaminating agents have to neutralize the free fluoric ions
- Calcium gluconate is used to rinse skin that has come into contact with hydrofluoric acid
- Using calcium gluconate at a 2% concentration results in the white corneal precipitates of insoluble CaF_2 or MgF_2 solids
- Anti-HF solution® is an effective amphoteric binder of the fluoride ion, keeping the cornea clear and decontaminated

After first aid rinsing
- Note clinical findings
- Effective first aid therapy can prevent long-term damage to eyes, even from highly corrosive agents
- Dua et al.[1] classification grades prognosis for the cornea, but the Reim classification (1997) grades the overall prognosis for the whole eye following injury

Clinical presentations of ocular burns

- Corneal erosion due to initial damage of the epithelium and later due to the lack of healing capacity of the epithelial layer dependent on limbal stem cell survival and activity
- Corneal opacity indicating reversible and in later stages irreversible damage of the corneal collagen glycoprotein matrix
- Ischaemia of the limbal vessel arcade, with healing deficiency expected in damage exceeding 60%
- Turbidity of lens and damage of iris are indicators of deep corrosive action and inflammatory response of the eye
- Conjunctival chemosis, indicating severe damage. Rinsing with hyperosmolar amphoteric solutions has resulted in a reduction in this symptom
- Conjunctival ischaemia is a more objective measure to evaluate the depth of damage of the conjunctiva and sclera

Prognosis of grading

Table 22.1 shows the prognosis for healing.

Table 22.1 Simple prognosis healing under the Dua classification of ocular burns

Grade I	Very good healing under therapy
Grade II-III	Good healing under therapy
Grade IV	Good to possible healing with surgical intervention
Grade V	Possible to poor healing with surgical intervention
Grade VI	Unlikely healing under therapy and surgical intervention

For the full grading system, see Dua HS, King AJ, Joseph A. A new classification of ocular surface burns. British Journal of Ophthalmology 2001;85(11):1379–83

Principles of medical treatment of ocular burns

- Improve corneal epithelial healing by lubrication with hyaluronic acid derivates
- Antibiotic protection, omitting macrolides (eg. gentamycin) and fluoroquinolones (ciprofloxacin) due to interference with epithelial healing
- Use steroids to inhibit the devastating autoimmune response and damage to stem cells
- Preservatives should be avoided as the high frequency of eye drops used cause damage to the surface of the eye
- Stop phosphate application on the eye as corneal calcification can occur

Proposed best practice

- Unpreserved hyaluronic acid lubricants
- Ointments of antibiotic and steroids, eg. Dexa-Polyspectrane®, Isopto Max®

Principles of surgical treatment of ocular burns

- Debridement of necrotic tissue under general anaesthetic
- Earliest surgical intervention is between 2 and 3 days after appropriate conservative treatment
- Residual conjunctival defects following necrosectomy can be successfully closed by tenonplasty, described by Teping et al.[2]
- Persistent corneal erosion following treatment with high dose steroids, lubricants, and antibiotic protection may warrant placement of an amniotic membrane graft combined with placement of a protective soft bandage lens
- Corneal grafts, autologous or homologous limbal stem cell grafts with systemic and local immune suppression as well as keratoprosthetic surgery should be considered for advanced stage burns of the orbit

These surgical approaches have a high risk of failure; however, when carried out meticulously in the hands of a specialist, these procedures can restore sight.

Further reading

Schrage NF, Struck HG, Gerard M. Recommendations for acute treatment for chemical and thermal burns of eyes and lids. Ophthalmology 2011;108(10):916–20.
Scott WJ, Schrage N, Dohlman C. Emergency eye rinse for chemical injuries: new considerations. JAMA Ophthalmol 2015;133(3):245.

References

1. Dua HS, King AJ, Joseph A. A new classification of ocular surface burns. British Journal of Ophthalmology 2001;85:1379–83.
2. Teping C, Reim M. Tenoplasty as a new surgical principle in the early treatment of the most severe chemical eye burns. Klinische Monatsblätter für Augenheilkunde 1989;194:1–5.

Hand burns

Introduction to hand burns

The hand only accounts for approximately 2–3% of the total body surface area (TBSA); however, it is rarely spared and thermal injury to the hand has consistently been shown to be a poor long-term outcome predictor. A comprehensive treatment plan must be formulated immediately following a thermal injury and continued through the recovery phase.

Thermally injured hand

- Accounts for over 75% of thermal injuries evaluated by the emergency medical system
- Scald injuries are common in the home, with children most likely to be injured
- Functional outcome is directly dependent on severity of initial injury and prevention of secondary injury (ie. compartment syndrome, desiccation of tendinous structures, nerves, etc.)
- Suspect abuse with well-defined dorsal contact thermal hand injures in children
- Acceptable outcomes can be expected with appropriately and timely management

Anatomy

- The hand consists of an anatomical component (hand) and a functional component (forearm)
- Must consider the hand in continuity with the forearm for optimal outcomes
- The anatomy of the hand predisposes the dorsum of the hand to more significant thermal injuries given the same heat transfer
- Dorsum of hand:
  - Non-glabellar skin is thin and mobile to allow for maximum joint mobility
  - Minimal distance between skin and extensor tendons increases the risk for complex involvement of deeper structures
- Volar/palmar hand:
  - Glabellar skin is thick and hairless thus more resistant to full thickness thermal injures
  - Only 15% of palmar injuries will require operative intervention

Hand function

Dependent on maintaining stability, range of motion, sensation, and power:

- Stability—avoidance of tendon desiccation and injury to the central extensor tendon is critical to avoid non-functional deformities (ie. Boutonniere deformity)
- Range of motion—50% of hand function is accomplished via the thumb. Maintenance of thumb length and function is critical to optimal hand outcome
- Power—maintenance of thumb and index allows for a functional pinch mechanism; handgrip power is dependent on maintaining function of middle, ring, and little fingers

Initial assessment

- History—evaluate mechanism of injury
- Initial assessment begins with a complete evaluation of the thermally injured individual
- Exclude electrical and chemical mechanisms
- ABCs—airway, breathing, and circulation must be stabilized prior to evaluation of the thermally injured hand
- Adequate fluid resuscitation is important to avoid vascular compromise; however, over-resuscitation may lead to interstitial oedema and vascular compromise

Burn wound evaluation

- Determine depth of injury: this will dictate conservative versus operative intervention
- Assess vascular integrity:
  - Capillary refill tested at fingernails
  - Allen's and digital Allen's test in unburnt skin
  - Monitor integrity with Doppler ultrasound to digit vessels or palmar arch
  - Monitor the five Ps—pain, pressure, pulselessness, paralysis, and paraesthesia frequently, as traditional signs of compartment syndrome may be absent. Inconclusive evaluation should lead to direct measure of compartmental pressures to avoid secondary injury to the hand. (Muscular injury can occur with prolonged forearm compartmental hypertension, 20–30 mmHg, and at lower thresholds in the hand)
- Assess for skeletal trauma:
  - Obtain appropriate radiographs
  - Maintain a high index of suspicion with industrial accidents

Estimation of hand surface area (rule of thumb)

A simple method of estimation of the burnt surface of a hand is to express the area involved in terms of the patient's thumbprint area (T) (see Table 23.1 and Fig. 23.1).
- Calculation of % TBSA = number of thumbprints ÷ 30
- One thumbprint (T) = 1/30th of 1% = 0.033% TBSA:
  - 3T burn = 0.1% TBSA

Table 23.1 Rule of thumb

Surface areas of the hand	Thumbprints (T)	% TBSA
Palm (excluding digits)	15	0.5
Dorsum (excluding digits)	15	0.5
Radial, ulnar palmar and dorsal aspects of each digit (20 surfaces)	2 on each surface, on each digit* (total 42)	0.066(1.4)
First web space	2	0.066
2nd, 3rd, 4th web spaces	1 on each space (total 3)	0.033(0.1)
Ulnar border of palm	3	0.1
Whole hand	80	2.66

*Volar surface of ring and middle finger 3T each.

Reproduced from Dargan D, Mandal A, Shokrollahi K Hand burns surface area: a rule of thumb. Burns (in press, March 2018) with permission from Elsevier.

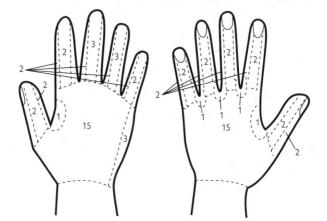

Fig. 23.1 Diagram of surface areas of the hand, showing estimated thumbprint (T) areas on each surface, including web spaces and radial/ulnar surfaces of digits.

Reproduced from Dargan D, Mandal A, Shokrollahi K. Hand burns surface area: a rule of thumb. Burns (in press, March 2018) with permission from Elsevier..

Initial management

- Burn wound: The concept of initial wound care consists of an aseptic and moist environment that can be easily assessed over time
- Burns to the hands can be initially managed by placing the hand/forearm in a clear plastic (polyethylene) bag, containing a mixture of a few millilitres each of chlorhexidine and liquid paraffin, which is then secured in place proximally
- This technique allows free mobilization of the hand and digits, and regular assessment of the burn wound

Prevent vascular compromise

- Constriction—extremity constriction may result from circumferential eschar, tight dressings, or oedema
- Thermal injures to the hands at risk of vascular compromise should be elevated to no more than 45° to minimize oedema, without impairing vascular inflow
- Avoid tight dressings via frequent evaluations by medical and/or nursing staff
- Circumferential upper limb burns with vascular compromise should be treated with urgent escharotomies/fasciotomies to avoid secondary injury (see Chapter 12)

Definitive treatment

Partial thickness burn

- Often heal with conservative management in less than 3 weeks and managed as outpatients
- Require all blisters debrided to ensure adequate burn wound assessment. One exception—small (<1–2 cm) volar intact blisters, with low suspicion for full thickness injury, may be debrided after 5–7 days to allow for epithelialization of the underlying tissue
- Appropriate dressings (see Chapter 17) without splints to allow full mobilization of all joints
- Physiotherapy and occupational therapy input is essential to improve outcomes

Deep partial thickness burn

- May heal over a longer period of time, but needs re-evaluating after 7–10 days, as may require excision and skin grafting

Full thickness burn

- All full thickness thermal injuries should be treated with prompt surgical intervention
- Studies have suggested that early surgical intervention in hand injuries reduces
  - Hospital stay
  - Cost
  - Time out of work
  - Hypertrophic scarring
- The goal is to re-establish hand mobility by 3 weeks
- All grafted thermal injures to the hand require an initial period of immobilization and evaluation in a functional position. This can be accomplished with splinting or K wire fixation of the interphalangeal joints and metacarpophalangeal joints
- Functional position:
  - Metacarpophalangeal joints 70–90° of flexion
  - Interphalangeal joints in extension
  - Wrist 20° of extension
  - Thumb abducted

Complex burns involving deep structures

- Exposure of neurovascular, tendinous, or bony structures may require vascularized coverage
- Consider neodermal products such as integra® followed by split thickness skin grafting, or local flaps versus pocketing techniques:
  - Dorsal hand injures—reverse radial forearm flap, groin flap
  - Dorsal hand and digital injuries—pocketing techniques into the ipsilateral abdominal wall versus thigh

Hand therapy

The majority of hand burns do not require surgical intervention. Occupational therapy and physiotherapy input is key to optimizing functional outcomes for many.

- Should form part of the initial assessment of a hand burn in a burns centre
- Encourage early range of motion exercises, with adequate analgesia
- Pressure garments for oedema management and pain control once burn dry
- Intermittent splintage for contracture management where necessary, eg. web space burns
- Detailed assessment of range of motion and targeted exercises, with review of progress
- Strengthening of muscles weakened by temporary disuse
- Functional assessment of daily activities and return to pre-morbid function, including use of household items
- Assistance with return to work

Outcomes

- The outcomes following thermal injuries to the hand are dependent on damage to the underlying structures, including the extensor tendons and joint capsules, and formation of contractures in the skin
- 75% of the incidence of future reconstructive procedures are for initial injures affecting underlying structures compared to 15% without
- Overall psychosocial functioning and re-integration has consistently been shown to be heavily dependent on hand function

Further reading

Luce EA. The acute and subacute management of the burned hand. Clinics in Plastic Surgery 2000;27:49–63.
Dargan D, Mandal A, Shokrollahi K. Hand burns surface area: a rule of thumb. Burns 2018;44;1346–51.

Perineal and genital burns

Causes of perineal and genital burns

Burns to the perineum and genitalia are most commonly encountered in the context of more widespread burns (occurring in <15% all patients sustaining burns). Isolated perineal/genital burns are uncommon, particularly in women, as the perineum is usually protected by surrounding anatomy and clothing. Adult burns are often due to liquid scalds and are usually relatively superficial, whereas flame burns are less common but often associated with more widespread leg/trunk burns and are usually more severe.

Particular challenges of perineal and genital burns

- Maintenance of wound hygiene in an area with high bacterial load (particularly coliforms)
- Consideration of need for urinary and/or faecal diversion
- Application and adherence of dressings
- Skin graft retention
- Scar contractures threatening genitourinary and sexual function, in addition to limiting leg movement
- Psychosexual sequelae
- Consideration of non-accidental injury

When encountered in children, isolated burns should raise concerns regarding non-accidental injury. Data from the USA indicated that 46–48% of isolated perineal and/or genital burns in children under 2 were non-accidental. Uniform depth burns with well-demarcated edges, perhaps in association with heel or foot scalds, are particularly suspicious for deliberate immersion injuries.

General principles for managing perineal and genital burns

- Meticulous hygiene
- Prevention of infection
- Conservative approach to surgical intervention

Initial management

Wound care

- Initially conservative with gauze debridement, cleansing, and topical antimicrobials/dressings
- Wounds allowed to fully demarcate prior to any excisional debridement
- Keeping thighs in ~15° abduction with a wedge may help prevent hip contractures

Urinary management

- The presence of perineal/genital burns should **not** automatically prompt urinary catheterization unless indicated
- Catheterization (per urethra or suprapubic) is indicated if required for monitoring burn resuscitation, if there is impending labial/penile oedema sufficient to cause urethral obstruction, or if pre-existing urinary incontinence (eg. in elderly patients) threatens wound hygiene
- Urethral catheterization may help prevent meatal stenosis
- Remove catheter at the earliest possible opportunity

Bowel management

- Prevention of faecal soiling is paramount to limit invasive wound infection, delayed wound healing, and graft loss
- Broadly speaking, there are four options:
  - Regular dressing changes and careful hygiene may suffice in continent and compliant patients
  - Induced constipation—*may* be appropriate in the short term. Few proponents as this risks overflow, bacterial translocation, etc. Low residue feed may be a better option to reduce stool frequency, but has nutritional implications
  - Faecal management tubes (±stool softeners)—most appropriate in sedated patients. Risks include mucosal ulceration and anal atony. Systems may bypass/leak
  - Temporary diverting colostomy—some proponents in young children or deep perineal burns. Risks include those of the procedure, parastomal hernia, and difficulties sealing stoma bags to burned abdominal wall

Delayed reconstruction

Perineum

- Most commonly cicatricial contracture between proximal inner thigh and perineum, or between genitalia and anus
- Reconstruction depends upon extent of scar and quality of adjacent tissues
- May enable excision and direct closure, or require local fasciocutaneous flaps (triangular/rhomboid/lotus), groin, or anterolateral thigh flaps

Male genitalia

- Extent of scarring may not be apparent in flaccid state
- If Buck's fascia spared, defects can be resurfaced with full thickness skin graft or split skin graft with dermal matrix
- If Buck's involved, defects require flap coverage
- Testicular burns are rare due to multiple layers of fascial coverage. If significant scrotal debridement necessitates flap coverage, muscle flaps may be less suitable as resultant higher testicular temperatures may influence spermatogenesis
- Requirement for penectomy and phalloplasty is thankfully very rare

Female genitalia

- Local skin flaps and grafts (±fat transfer) can be used for labial reconstruction
- Larger defects require flap reconstruction
- Vaginal and introital stenosis may limit options for normal vaginal delivery

Further reading

Angel C, Shu T, French D, et al. Genital and perineal burns in children: 10 years of experience at a major burn center. Journal of Pediatric Surgery 2002;37:99.

Bordes J, Le Floch R, Bourdais L, et al. Perineal burn care: French working group recommendations. Burns 2014;40:655.

Michielsen DP, Lafaire C. Management of genital burns: a review. International Journal of Urology 2010;17:755.

Skin substitutes

Purpose and development of skin substitutes

Skin substitutes are a heterogeneous group of wound coverage materials that aid in would closure and replace the functions of the skin. They were developed as an adjunct or alternative to autografts, which remain the current gold standard for the treatment of burns.

Advantages of skin substitutes

- Provide immediate wound cover—temporary or permanent
- Mechanical barrier to infection and fluid loss
- Optimize conditions for healing and keep the wound bed moist
- Stimulate the wound bed and promote new tissue growth/provide a neodermal base
- Can minimize scar contraction
- Available in large quantities

Disadvantages of skin substitutes

- Expensive
- Can be difficult to store with short half-life
- Learning curve for clinical application and use
- Ethical issues may limit their use in certain religious groups
- Risk of cross-infection (potentially with allografts and xenografts)

Skin substitutes for temporary wound cover

Biobrane
Dow–Hickham, Sugarland, TX, USA.

Type
Temporary biosynthetic dressing.

Features
- Bilaminate membrane composed of a thin outer silicone membrane (epidermal analogue) with a knitted nylon mesh
- Porcine type 1 collagen is incorporated into the silicone and nylon components
- The chemically bonded collagen promotes adherence to the burn wound with a fibrin bond
- The semipermeable membrane allows drainage of exudate from the wound surface
- Prevents evaporative fluid loss and the development of infection

Applications
- Temporary coverage for partial thickness burns that are expected to heal within 14 days. The dressing adheres to the wound and detaches as the burn heals
- Temporary coverage for freshly excised full-thickness wounds
- Donor site coverage
- TENS (toxic epidermal necrolysis)

Advantages
- Can obviate painful dressing changes, reduce inpatient treatment and length of stay in partial thickness burns
- Pain relief and accelerated healing when used to cover donor sites
- Specific anatomical designs available, eg. gloves

Drawbacks
- Non-adherence to the burn wound can lead to accumulation of fluid and subsequent infection. Any fluid accumulations and infection should be released
- Staphylococcal toxic shock syndrome in children from pooling of exudate underneath the dressing has been reported

TransCyte (formerly Dermagraft)
Advanced Tissue Sciences, La Jolla, CA, USA.

Type
Temporary biosynthetic dressing.

Composition
- Consists of a polymer membrane and neonatal human fibroblasts cultured on a nylon mesh in vitro. Prior to cell growth, the nylon mesh is coated with porcine dermal collagen and bonded to a silicon membrane
- The fibroblasts proliferate within the nylon mesh during the manufacturing process and secrete dermal collagen, growth factors,

glycosaminoglycans (GAGs), and fibronectin to aid wound healing. Cryopreservation renders the fibroblasts non-viable

Applications
- Temporary covering for excised full thickness burns prior to autografting
- Temporary coverage for partial thickness burns that do not require autografting. The dressing adheres to the wound and detaches as the burn heals
- Partial-thickness facial burns: the pliable dressing easily conforms, rapidly adheres and integrates to protect the wound. Decreased pain, accelerated epithelialization, and healing over conventional topical therapies has been suggested

Drawbacks
- Cumbersome storage and pre-use preparation: stored frozen between –70°C and –20°C and can be thawed no longer than 2 hours before use. If stored correctly, it has a shelf life of 18 months
- More expensive than biobrane but no real benefit has been demonstrated over Biobrane in partial thickness burns

Allograft

Type
Cryopreserved cadaver skin.

Features
- Second choice following autograft
- Takes readily and provides durable coverage

Applications
- Definitive closure with the allograft–autograft sandwich technique: widely meshed autograft covers the wound bed to provide permanent closure. An allograft (2:1 mesh) is laid over the autograft to provide a temporary protective physiological barrier
- Estimating usage: 0.5 cm^2 allograft/cm^2 burns <40% TBSA, and 1.82 cm^2 allograft/cm^2 burn for 40–80% TBSA
- Temporary biological dressing for donor sites, allowing them to heal prior to reharvesting

Drawbacks
- Expensive
- Requires storage at –40 to –80°C
- Cryopreservation decreases viability by 54% to 73% of fresh tissue
- Poor barrier function
- Risk of disease transmission despite screening of tissue donors and testing for bacterial and viral contamination

Skin substitutes for wound closure

Alloderm
LifeCell Corporation, Branchburg, NJ, USA.

Type
Cryopreserved acellular dermal allograft.

Features
- Split-thickness skin grafts are obtained from human cadavers (the donors are screened for transmissible diseases)
- The epithelial components and dermal cellular components are removed, the residual dermis is treated with a proprietary detergent to inactivate viruses, and then cryopreserved
- Provides a non-antigenic upper dermal scaffold consisting of basement membrane proteins and type IV and VII collagen
- Available in a variety of thicknesses
- Rehydrated in a sterile saline solution immediately before use
- Following application to a wound bed, it is repopulated by host cells, revascularized and incorporated into the tissue. It functions as a template for dermal regeneration

Applications
- Thin layer of alloderm is used to cover acutely excised burn wounds or incisional releases in combination with simultaneous placement of an overlying thin, split-thickness autograft

Advantages
- Reported to have good 'take' rates
- When compared with the use of split-thickness autograft alone for full-thickness wounds, it is thought to result in less scarring and to provide more pliable soft tissue cover

Drawbacks
- Expensive
- Relatively marginal benefit

Integra
Integra LifeSciences, Plainsboro, NJ, USA

Type
Dermal analogue.

Features
- Bi-laminar structure
- Superficial layer of fenestrated silicone membrane provides a temporary epidermal barrier function, and protection against fluid loss and bacterial colonization
- Deep layer composed of cross-linked bovine collagen and chondroitin-6-sulphate, provides a biodegradable framework
- Once applied to the wound, the deep collagen layer promotes the migration of fibroblasts and endothelial cells and becomes

bio-integrated in the wound. A vascular neodermis is formed in approximately 2–3 weeks
- After integration 2–3 weeks later, the silastic layer is removed and an ultrathin split-thickness skin graft is applied in the second stage

Applications
- Commonly used to provide immediate cover in the treatment of major burn where a paucity of available donor area precludes early autografting. Frequent thin, split-thickness grafts can be reharvested for staged reconstruction in extensive burns
- Used for burn contracture release
- Pliable soft tissue cover over joints and tendons where flaps may be too complex and bulky, and skin grafts alone would provide poor aesthetic and functional result
- Integra may provide a well-vascularized neodermis and allow skin autografting without the need for complex reconstruction where there is poorly vascularized tissue with exposure of bone, cartilage, or tendons
- Integra combined with VAC therapy may accelerate integration and vascularization, shorten the time between the first and second stages, reduce length of hospital stay, minimize dressing changes and remove fluid from under the matrix sheet

Advantages
- Long shelf-life
- Available in large amounts without any preparation
- Can provide thin soft tissue cover without the bulk of a flap
- Allows good functional and aesthetic result compared to split skin graft alone
- May provide a more durable and superior long-term aesthetic result with less hypertrophic scarring and pruritus compared to those burns treated by conventional excision and grafting alone

Drawbacks
- Requires a two-stage procedure and extended hospital stay
- Time-consuming dressing changes required until healing is complete
- Dermal matrix 'take' can be poor and become infected
- Haematoma or seroma can accumulate under the matrix
- Steep learning curve
- Expensive

Matriderm

Skin and Health Care AG, Billerbeck, Germany.

Type

Bovine dermal substitute features
- Structurally intact matrix of bovine type I collagen with elastin
- Matrix serves as a support structure for in growth of cells and vessels
- Elastin component improves the stability and elasticity of the regenerating tissue. As the healing process advances, fibroblast lays down the extracellular matrix and the matrix resorbs

Applications
- Useful in functional areas, eg. over joints and tendons, where elasticity, pliability and stability is desirable
- Can provide a thin, pliable, and aesthetic pleasing skin cover

Advantages
- Allows one-stage reconstruction with synchronous application of dermal substitutes and skin grafts
- Thought to reduce wound contracture and increase elasticity of skin and provide a more pliable and durable skin cover than using a skin graft alone
- As reconstruction is a single stage, there is less risk of infection, fewer dressing changes and potentially shorter hospital stay required compared to that of Integra
- Available in 1 mm and 2 mm thickness, in various sizes

Drawbacks
- Expensive.

Apligraf (Graftskin)
Organogenesis, Canton, MA, USA.

Type
Bi-layered living skin equivalent.

Features
- Engineered collagen-based substitute containing viable cells
- Designed to mimic the structure of the human skin
- Bi-layered: the superficial layer consists of a cornified epidermal layer of neonatal allogeneic keratinocytes and the deep layer (dermal analogue) combines living neonatal allogeneic fibroblasts in a gel of type I bovine collagen
- Not attached to any polymer membrane

Applications
- Can be used as a temporary covering over meshed expanded autograft for excised burn wounds

Advantages
- Apligraf combined with autograft is thought to produce more favourable results than autograft only with more pliable soft tissue cover, less scar formation, pigmentation, and improved texture of the graft

Drawbacks
- Currently the most sophisticated and most expensive commercially available tissue-engineered product
- The material is supplied to a given date and has to be applied 'fresh'
- Requires careful handling and short-term storage: shelf-life of just 5 days at room temperature to ensure viability of the cells in the two layers

Cultured epithelial autograft (CEA)

Features

Sheets

- Requires a full thickness skin biopsy of several square centimetres: a 2 cm^2 biopsy produces a 1.8 m^2 confluent sheet five cells thick
- The sheets of epithelial cells, about six cells thick, are attached to a petroleum-impregnated gauze carrier to facilitate the physical handling of the otherwise extremely fragile, thin sheets
- 3 weeks' preparation time

Suspension

- Fibrin glue suspension takes less time to process but cells are less mature
- Used either in combination with widely meshed split skin graft or for donor-site re-epithelialization

Advantages

- Autologous cells
- Only a small biopsy needed

Disadvantages

- Expensive
- Long preparation time of 3–5 weeks
- Provides very thin and fragile skin cover and the resulting epithelium is unstable. Although initial graft take is good, there may be late graft loss with spontaneous blistering and infection many months after grafting
- The skin graft may be more susceptible to infection and contractures
- A high degree of coordination is required between the burn unit and laboratory to use the cultured epithelial autograft sheets at their optimum

Further reading

Jansen LA, De Caigny P, Guay NA, et al. The evidence base for the acellular dermal matrix AlloDerm: a systematic review. Annals of Plastic Surgery 2013;70:587–94.

Nicoli, F, Rampinelli, I, Godwin, Y. The application of Integra in a challenging context. Scars, Burns & Healing 2016;2:2059513116672789.

Pham C, Greenwood J, Cleland H, Woodruff P, Maddern G. Bioengineered skin substitutes for the management of burns: a systematic review. Burns 2007;33:946–57.

Occupational and physiotherapy

Occupational therapy

Burns as a specialty demands occupational therapy skills and experience drawn from a variety of clinical areas, ranging from musculoskeletal through to mental health, and covers both in-patient and out-patient care simultaneously. As part of the wider burns MDT, the occupational therapist is involved in the treatment of a patient from injury through to scar maturation, or until adulthood in the case of paediatric patients.

The core values and beliefs of occupational therapy are epitomized within the field of burns. Patient treatment is based upon a wide range of different methods and theories focused around a biopsychosocial model, where promoting independence and enhancing function is the central aim of therapeutic engagement. The diversity of injury and the subsequent consequences that can affect the patient are wide-ranging. Therefore, a unique approach to each patient to address their needs, encourage function and ultimately fulfil realistic goals as individuals is key.

The occupational therapy role

Occupational therapy begins on admission to a burn ward or intensive care, and continues long after discharge. Most of the treatment modalities employed are used within both in-patient and out-patient care.

Treatments and interventions:

- Splinting
  - To prevent joint/soft tissue and scar contractures
  - Protect graft sites
  - Increase range of movement (ROM)
  - Improve function
  - Compensatory movement splints to encourage or allow normal movement including dynamic splinting
- Positioning
  - To prevent graft/scar contractures
- Functional rehabilitation
  - Aim to increase independence in activities of daily living (ADLs)
  - ROM and strengthening exercises centred around activity, eg. facilitating ADLs, workshop, play
  - Graded activity including some assisted activity
  - Use of some compensatory techniques either temporary or permanent, eg adapted cutlery, custom-made adaptations
  - Specialized upper limb rehab using task simulation equipment
  - Mental and cognitive stimulation activities to enhance mood and thought processes
- Wheelchair assessment and provision
- Discharge planning
  - Identification of appropriate discharge destination
  - Equipment provision and minor adaptations to home
  - Home visits
  - Liaison with social worker and identification of care needs.
- Social re-integration, life readjustment, and psychological support, eg. supporting and facilitating leaving safe ward environment, and coping with reactions to injury
- Scar management—to begin as soon as clinically possible to gain optimum results
  - Encourage normal movement and use of body to minimize contractures
  - Application of pressure garments
  - Use of silicone gels and conformers
  - Massage
  - Splinting: to prevent contracture, stretch existing scar, or serial splinting
  - Cosmetic camouflage
  - Referral onto other agencies, eg. orthotics, maxillofacial
  - Outreach

- Return to work/life roles
  - Includes heavy rehabilitation programmes as an out-patient
  - Work place/school visits
  - Liaising with employers and schools to ensure correct levels of support are in place to maximize patient independence and encourage job retention
  - Support with redeployment where necessary
  - Referral onto relevant external agencies

Physiotherapy

The survival rate of major burns has improved with recent advances in care resulting in more complex rehabilitation needs. All burns, irrespective of severity, have the potential to affect people physically and emotionally and the physiotherapists' role within the multidisciplinary team is to ensure as good an outcome as possible in terms of movement, strength, function, and aesthetics.

The physiotherapist will be involved with the burn-injured patient both as an inpatient and an outpatient and will address the following aspects of care as applicable to individual patient's needs.

This chapter has been written in accordance with the British Burns Association Therapy Standards[1] and it is assumed that individuals will work within the boundaries of their professional body and knowledge. It is imperative that burns patients are managed by experienced therapists who are regularly involved in the care of these patients.

- The aims of physiotherapy intervention are to
  - Maintain respiratory function
  - Manage oedema
  - Assist in management of pain, itch and sensation
  - Maintain joint range of motion
  - Maintain cardiovascular fitness/strength
  - Aid functional independence
  - Scarring
  - Provide psychological support

The extent of physiotherapy intervention that is required is dependent upon the extent/depth of the injury, the surgery required and patients' individual needs.

For a greater depth of understanding of the physiotherapists role within the care of the burn-injured patient the British Burns Association Therapy Standards[1] can be reviewed.

The physiotherapy role

Respiratory function
- The aims of physiotherapy interventions are to
  - Maintain clear airways
  - Remove excess secretions
  - Improve gaseous exchange
  - Prevent and treat atelectasis
- Physiotherapeutic interventions to aid respiratory function are
  - Education
  - Mobility
  - Breathing exercises
  - Chest manual techniques
  - Humidification of oxygen
  - Suction via a nasal or oral airway
  - Positioning to aid drainage and/or gaseous exchange
  - Continuous positive airways pressure (CPAP)
  - Intermittent positive pressure breathing (IPPB)
  - Tracheostomy management

Manage oedema
Oedema control will prevent later complications of soft tissue adherence and loss of joint range of motion. This is especially important with hand burns but applies to all areas of the body. Techniques that aid oedema control are
- Elevation
- Positioning
- Massage
- Compression
- Active exercise

Assist in management of pain, itch, and sensation
Pain can be a significant issue during physiotherapy treatment sessions for a burn-injured patient. Analgesia is crucial to promote patient involvement and compliance. In addition to pharmacological management the physio-therapist can assist in pain control and later both itch and sensory disturbance can be addressed with therapy interventions.

Techniques that aid management of pain, itch and sensation are:
- Entonox
- Education, reassurance and distraction
- Splinting
- Exercise
- Massage
- Sensory re-education/desensitization

Maintain joint range of motion

Skin contractures at specific anatomical sites are inevitable following burn injury, eg. anterior/posterior axillary folds. The physiotherapist will use therapy interventions to limit these skin contractures and prevent them developing into joint contractures where the joint structures (capsule, ligaments etc.) also become shortened and restrict joint range of motion.

Range of movement exercises are started as soon as possible following a burn injury then adapted appropriately following surgical intervention.

Interventions

Positioning

The patient's joints are positioned in anti-contracture postures between exercise sessions to maintain soft tissue length. This can be achieved using static splints or by advising on resting postures. It is important that the whole team, relatives, and the patient are aware of optimal positioning to maximize compliance.

Active exercises

This involves the patient actively moving their joints through full range of motion. Active motion is the ideal therapeutic intervention as it maintains soft tissue extensibility, maintains muscle strength, creates a muscle pump to reduce oedema, maintains normal sensory motor feedback, and promotes independence. An individual exercise programme should be developed for the specific needs of each patient.

Passive exercises

This involves the physiotherapist moving the patient's joints through normal physiological range. This is necessary if the patient is ventilated or unable to exercise independently due to lack of strength/nerve palsy/compliance. It is useful for the physiotherapist to go into theatre when the patient is anaesthetized so range of movement can be assessed and stretches performed without any distress to the patient.

Maintain cardiovascular fitness/strength

The longevity of burn care management plus the systemic effects of burn injury will cause a reduction in cardiovascular fitness and strength. The physiotherapist will endeavour to maintain the patients' fitness and strength during the acute stages of their injury and regain their previous level of fitness/strength to as near normal as possible during the later stages of rehabilitation.

Techniques that aid cardiovascular fitness/strength are
- Mobility
- Active exercise
- Strengthening
- Optimization of cardio fitness
- Education to patients and their family
- Resistive exercise
- Functional exercise
- Proprioceptive neuromuscular facilitation

Scarring

Alongside the occupational therapists, physiotherapists will assist in the management of scarring. See the Occupational therapy section.

Aid functional independence

The ultimate aim of physiotherapy intervention is to return the patient to as near normal function as possible. This will involve rehabilitation of mobility, range of motion, strength/endurance, social re-integration, and functional independence as soon as possible to enable patients to regain their former life. A multidisciplinary approach (including family and friends) to this is essential throughout their recovery to ensure consistency.

Psychological support

Alongside the rest of the team the burns physiotherapist is in an ideal position to develop a rapport with the patient and to identify/address their psychosocial needs. The use of agreed/achievable goal setting as a motivational tool during their rehabilitation can support their psychological recovery. A multidisciplinary approach (including family and friends) to this is essential throughout their recovery to ensure consistency.

Reference

1. British Burns Association. Standards of physiotherapy and occupational therapy practice in the management of burn injured adults and children. London: British Burns Association 2017.

Chapter 27

Outcome measures for burns

Introduction to outcome measures for burns

Advances in burn care have markedly reduced mortality rates in the acute phase. As patients survive longer, a variety of measures of outcomes beyond mortality, such as function and quality of life, have been developed. Such standardized outcome measures allow treatments to be compared and are useful in monitoring response to therapy. They also allow comparison of outcomes between centres. Certain outcome measures are aggregated into scales while others are considered separately. This chapter does not include all published measures but lists only those validated or most commonly used for burns patients.

Classification

There are various ways of classifying burns outcome measures (BOMs). BOMs are used to evaluate short- and long-term (see Table 27.1) outcomes. Some measures may apply to more than one time-point.

Apart from the obvious physical effects (Table 27.2), the incidence of psychosocial morbidity such as post-traumatic stress disorder (PTSD), depression, social isolation, and perceived low-quality of life in burn survivors is high. Several measures exist to ascertain the degree of such morbidity in burns patients (Table 27.3). Some scales measure more than one domain, eg. the SF-36 assesses biological, psychological, and social functioning. There are also measures developed specifically for children as their experience is unique and distinct from adult survivors (Table 27.4). Some scales measure outcomes in limbs (Table 27.5) and others outcomes are usually regarded on their own (Table 27.6).

Table 27.1 Examples of outcome measures relevant to different time-points

Short-term	Mortality, length of stay (LOS), determinants of the hypermetabolic state, biochemical, and physiological markers for morbidity assessment
Long-term	Functional scores: eg. exercise tolerance and grip strength, functional independence measure, functional assessment for burns
	Quality of life scales: eg. short form 36 (SF-36), Vineland Adaptive Behaviour Scales Survey Form (VABS-SF)
	Scar Assessment scales: Vancouver, Seattle and Hamilton Scar Scales, Patient and Observer Scar Assessment Scale
	Psychosocial outcome scales: eg. Coping with Burns Questionnaire, Satisfaction With Appearance Scale, Burn Specific Health Scale, Burn Specific Pain Anxiety Scale, Health Outcomes Burn Questionnaire

Table 27.2 Biological/physical outcome measures

Outcome measure(s)	Explanation and features
Determinants of burn injury hypermetabolic response: (heart rate, core temperature; organ function; body composition (lean muscle mass, bone mineral content by dual image X-ray absorptiometry), resting energy expenditure (Harris Bennedict formula), stable isotope tracers)	Burn patients are hypermetabolic up to 2 years post-injury. This state diminishes lean body mass, weakens muscles, and is associated with poor immune function and wound healing. It is characterized by increased energy expenditure, raised temperature, and increased protein, fat and glycogen breakdown. β-blockers, oxandrolone, growth hormone and insulin are all modulators of the hypermetabolic response. These outcome measures can be used to monitor return to normal metabolic state and also as research tools
Vancouver Scar Scale (VSS)	Aims to standardize assessments of scar height, pigmentation, vascularity, and pliability between assessors. This scale is widely used but is not considered reliable unless used by at least three assessors. A modified VSS also assesses pain and pruritus. Dermatospectrometry, chromametry, durometry, planimetry, and histologic micrometry can all be used to provide objective readings of aspects of the VSS.
Seattle Scar Scale (SSS)	Uses the scar surface, thickness, border height, and pigmentation differences between scar and adjacent normal skin to describe the general appearance of a scar. May be more appropriate for patients with widespread burns whereas the VSS selects a scar of 4 cm^2 or less. It is unreliable for comparing cosmetic outcomes. A modification is the Matching Assessment of Scars and Photograph (MASP) tool which uses a gridded body map to help relocate the scar at subsequent assessment. Itch can also be assessed using the Questionnaire For Pruritus Assessment
Hamilton Scar Scale (HSS)	Assesses scar height, vascularity, pigmentation, and irregularity from photographs
Patient and Observer Scar Assessment Scale (POSAS)	Although this scale measures the same parameters as the VSS, SSS, and HSS, it has the advantage of including a patient-rated component. Some authors suggest this may be the best tool
Functional Independence Measure (FIM)	The FIM was not developed specifically for burns patients but can be used mainly to predict the need for rehabilitation, and therefore may be more useful as a discharge planning tool
Functional Assessment for Burns (FAB)	Assesses patients' ability to independently feed, wash, dress, transfer, walk, climb stairs, and use toilets. The FAB is similar to the FIM but does not assess communication, continence, psychosocial interaction, and cognition. Also, the FAB measures a patient's ability to complete 100% of an activity whereas the FIM assesses components of activities

Table 27.3 Psychosocial outcome measures

Outcome measure(s)	Explanation and features
Burn Specific Health Scale (BSHS)	The BSHS is a comprehensive 114-item constructed by combining burn-specific questions with the Sickness Impact Profile, Index of Activities of Daily Living, and the General Well-being Schedule. It is used to measure the quality of life of burn survivors. Several variations of the BSHS have been formulated. The most commonly used is the BSHS-Brief, which has proven to be effective in different countries
Satisfaction With appearance Scale (SWAP)	A 14-item questionnaire developed and validated to assess the subjective appraisal and social-behavioural components of body image in burns survivors. Six of the items were adapted from the BSHS
Coping With Burns Questionnaire (CWBQ)	A 33-item measure of coping mechanisms after burns and associated trauma. Patients are assessed on emotional support, problem solving, avoidance, adjustment, self-control, and instrumental action. As patients are asked to think back to the time they were discharged, there may be a degree of recall bias
SF-36	A 36-item measure of quality of life not developed specifically for burns patients but validated. Measures global reintegration and socialization under eight equally weighted domains: general health and perceptions of, vitality, physical and pain, physical role function, emotional role function, social role function, and mental health
Burn-Specific Pain Anxiety Scale (BSPAS)	A useful marker for patients who might be at risk of diminished function post-discharge. A five-item abbreviated version has also been validated for burns patients. It is, however, validated only for in-patients
Beck Depression Inventory (BDI) and Hospital Anxiety and Depression Scale (HADS)	Both the 21-item BDI-II and 14-item HADS have been used as measures of depression in burns patients. The BDI-II assesses both physical and emotional symptoms of depression while the HADS was developed as a screening tool for anxiety and depression. Caution should be practised when interpreting the results of these scales as some authors have noted that disturbances in some items from the scale such as sleep, libido and appetite could be due to the physical injury itself
Impact of Events Scale (IES)	The original 15-item IES patient-reported scale rates patients' experiences of two cardinal features of PTSD: intrusion and avoidance. Other measures that have been used to assess frequency and severity of PTSD stigmata in burns patients include the Davidson Trauma Scale

(Continued)

Table 27.3 (Contd.)

Outcome measure(s)	Explanation and features
Impact of Event-Scale (IES)	The original 15-item score comprises two subscales assessing intrusion and avoidance symptoms. A revision (IES-R) was designed to include hyperarousal symptoms. Both the original and revised versions are self-report instruments for symptoms of PTSD. The IES-R is a good screening tool for PTSD and can identify patients with subsyndromal PTSD 1 year after burn injury
Perceived Stigmatisation Questionnaire (PSQ)	This scale measures the frequency of various behaviours from other people which stigmatize burn survivors. These behaviours include staring, avoidance, confusion, rudeness, bullying, and pressurizing burn survivors to alter their appearance. It has been validated for use in both adult and paediatric burn survivors
Social Comforts Questionnaire (SCQ)	This scale was developed concurrently with the PSQ. It aims to measure perceived social isolation and the invasion of privacy

Table 27.4 Paediatric-specific burn outcome measures

Outcome measure(s)	Explanation and features
VABS-SF	These scales are designed to measure children's typical performance with regards to communication, daily living skills, socialization, and motor skills and NOT their ability
Health Outcomes Burn Questionnaire (HOBQ)	A quality-of-life measure for children. Versions exist for children 5 years and younger and from 6 to 18 years. Assesses parents' opinions on the child's play, language, gross and fine motor skills, family, behaviour, pain and itching, appearance, satisfaction, and concerns

Table 27.5 Limb outcome measures

Outcome measure(s)	Explanation and features
Lower limb	The single leg stance, tandem walk, and timed up-and-go tests are validated for burns patients, as is the BSHS-B. Other lower limb function measures such as the Lower Limb Functional Index have not been validated for burns
Upper limb	These include the Michigan Hand Outcomes Questionnaire an abbreviated 11-item version of the Disability of the Arm Shoulder and Hand (quickDASH) symptom scale are validated for use in burns patients

Table 27.6 Single variable outcome measures

Outcome measure(s)	Explanation and features
Mortality rate	Number of deaths per unit time. Most valuable for measuring acute phase outcomes
Pain	Can be measured using several tools such as the visual analogue scale, McGill Pain Questionnaire and the Brief Pain Inventory (BPI). The BPI is a comprehensive tool but has not been widely adopted by burns carers
Length of stay	Indicates burns-associated morbidity and cost of treatment. May be more accurate if measured retrospectively accounting for mistimed discharge, eg. patient is readmitted within days of discharge
Range of movement (ROM)	A marker for joint mobility. Goniometry and linear measurements are validated measures for ROM
Wound infection	Can be diagnosed by biopsy, culture, tissue histology and other subjective stigmata of infection (pain, redness, odour, and systemic symptoms)
Exercise tolerance, grip strength	These assess return to pre-injury activity level by measuring muscle strength and for exercise tolerance, aerobic capacity. Strength can be measured using free weights or dynamometry. An exercise tolerance test using the modified Bruce protocol is often used to measure aerobic capacity
Return to work	An indirect indicator of a patient's ability to reintegrate into society

Further reading

Pereira C, Murphy K, Herndon D. Outcome measures in burn care. Is mortality dead? Burns. 2004;30(8):761–71.

https://www.britishburnassociation.org/downloads/BBA_Outcomes_Doc_2nd_Edition.pdf

Falder S, Browne Aa, Eedgar D, Staples Ee, Fong J, Rrea S, Wood F. Core outcomes for adult burn survivors: a clinical overview. Burns. 2009;35(5):618–41.

Burns scar management

Common types of burn scars and interventions

For almost all burns scars, avoidance of exposure to sunlight, high factor sun screen for at least 2 years, and massage with suitable moisturizer is generally recommended.

Hypertrophic and keloid scars

Hypertrophic scars are erythematous, raised, and itchy. Keloid scars tend to be of a greater order of severity and extend beyond the boundaries of the original scar/injury.

Interventions

- Pressure therapy (pressure garments or masks)
- Silicone therapy
- Massage
- Intralesional corticosteroids
- Laser treatment (see Chapter 44)
- Moisturizers including medicated ones to help with itch and hydration

Keloids only: also
- Intralesional 5-fluorouracil
- Intralesional cryotherapy
- Brachytherapy and radiotherapy
- Surgery (last resort due to high recurrence, and often combined with other modalities)

Intralesional corticosteroids such as triamcinolone are one of the most successful and safe interventions for those that respond. In general, most other interventions tend to be for 'steroid non-responsive' cases.

Scar contractures (see also Chapter 30)
- Surgical scar release: skin grafts, reconstructive flaps, dermal substitutes (see Chapter 25)
- Laser treatment (mild)
- Splintage (prevention is better than cure)

Common scar interventions such as corticosteroid injections have limited success in mature scar contractures which do not have a hypertrophic element.

Mature scars

These are non-hypertrophic scars which will neither improve nor worsen spontaneously.

They will be of cosmetic concern and often cause functional limitation.
- Cosmetic camouflage
- Massage including interventions such as vacuum massage systems
- Laser (colour, contour, camouflage ability)
- Surgery and other interventions for functional and/or cosmetic limitations

Common scar interventions such as corticosteroid injections have limited success in mature scars.

Hyperpigmented scars

These scars show discolouration which is different from erythema (both may co-exist).

- Laser
- Dermabrasion
- Cosmetic camouflage
- Hydroquinone-based topical treatments (limited success)

Hypopigmented scars

- Cosmetic camouflage is the mainstay of treatment as reintroducing pigmentation is challenging and has highly variable and inconsistent results from most modalities available including:
  - Laser or dermabrasion with or without autologous cell transfer (eg. Re-Cell)
  - Micropigmentation and tattooing

Iatrogenic and surgical scars

Iatrogenic scars in burns are usually donor sites from split thickness skin grafts (STSGs) and full thickness skin grafts (FTSGs).

These scars may be amenable to a range of interventions to improve them as described before depending on the problems (eg. vascular laser for erythema, silicone and pressure for early hypertrophic scars).

Other iatrogenic changes are most frequently from corticosteroid injections, causing erythema, telangiectasia, and atrophy. Combined vascular (pulsed dye and/or Nd:YAG) is the mainstay of treatment for this problem.

Novel interventions for burn scars

- Platelet-rich plasma
- Autologous fat grafting
- Photodynamic therapy
- Tissue mechano-stimulation (LPG-Endermologie/'vacuum massage')

The holistic management of scars including psychological support is paramount.

Further reading

Alser OH, Goutos I. The evidence behind the use of platelet-rich plasma (PRP) in scar management: a literature review. Scars, Burns & Healing 2018;4:2059513118808773.

Goutos I, Ogawa R. Brachytherapy in the adjuvant management of keloid scars: literature review. Scars, Burns & Healing 2017;3:2059513117735483.

Riyat H, Touil L, Briggs M, Shokrollahi K. Autologous fat grafting for scars, healing and pain: a review. Scars, Burns & Healing 2017;3:2059513117728200.

Shokrollahi K (ed.). Laser management of scars. Springer-Nature, 2019.

Shokrollahi K, Whitaker IS, Nahai F. Flaps: practical reconstructive surgery. Stuttgart: Thieme, 2017.

Yeates R, Rospigliosi E, Thompson AR. A mixed methods evaluation of medical tattooing for people who have experienced a burn injury. Scars, Burns & Healing 2018;4:2059513118784721.

Principles of burn reconstruction

Key principles

Burn reconstruction starts with the initial surgery and continues until either the maximal functional and aesthetic outcome has been achieved, or the patient and/or surgeon feel that no further intervention is warranted. Communication and understanding of the limitations of surgery are essential to ensure that the appropriate approach is taken. While reconstruction is considered to be surgical, it is important not to forget the other contributing modalities that are essential to address the specific needs of the post-burn patient, such as splinting, physiotherapy, camouflage, laser, and scar management. In the ideal situation there should be a specialist, integrated team able to assess and plan a treatment programme dependent on the needs and wishes of the patient and the expertise and skills of the burn reconstruction team. Successful burn reconstruction owes much to effective early burn care and the prevention of complex scar contracture sequelae. Early excision and grafting of deep burns, coupled with carefully constructed regimes of splinting, scar therapy, and mobilization, has done much to reduce post-burn contractures and hypertrophic scarring, but there is still the need for surgical reconstructive procedures (both simple and complex) in certain cases. In countries where there are delays in initial treatment, minimal excision and grafting, and a lack or total absence of rehabilitation, the needs for functional surgical reconstruction are much higher.

Principles of reconstruction can be considered in terms of assessment and timing.

Assessment

Consider the 5 Ps

Problems
- Physical
  - Consider: Where are the scars, are they limiting function, are they clearly visible, are they painful, do they itch, are there areas of breakdown, what is it that bothers the patient etc.?
- Psychological
  - Consider: Is the problem more of perception, are there underlying social and psychological or relationship issues etc.?

Priorities

The priorities need to be considered from both the surgeon's point of view and the patient's as these are not necessarily the same, in which case the issues need to be carefully explored and discussed. From the surgical perspective, the priorities can be classified as urgent or non-urgent. Urgent indications would include severe ectropion leading to corneal exposure, severe microstomia, neck synechia limiting ventilation, and areas of unhealed or ulcerating scar (especially if long term where there is a risk of SCC formation). Non-urgent procedures still need to be prioritized and this depends on each individual patient. Sometimes it is better to do a small simple procedure first, other times it is better to address a more major contracture, but in general functional improvement takes priority over purely aesthetic improvement.

Possibilities

When considering the possibilities, it is important to think of both surgical and non-surgical options. Within surgical options, all the possibilities should be considered and rather than progressing stepwise using the 'reconstructive ladder' (starting with the most simple technique and moving up to the most advanced), the most appropriate should be chosen. It is not about what 'could' be done, but what 'should' be done. Within the surgical toolbox there are many different options and the first decision with respect to scar contractures is whether to do an *incisional* or *excisional* release (ie. whether to cut through the scar or cut out the scar). Then all the options for providing skin ± soft tissue cover need to be considered and this will include direct closure, local flaps, split and full thickness skin grafts, composite grafts, tissue expansion, free tissue transfer, and use of dermal templates.

Patient perceptions

It is critical that the patient has a realistic understanding of what can be achieved and what cannot be achieved. Good, clear communication is essential and the length of surgery, likely hospital stay, time off work, postoperative physiotherapy, splinting, scar management, etc., need to be understood by the patient as the rehabilitation investment can be quite considerable and this needs to be weighed against the likely improvement achieved.

Plan of action
Once the above process has been gone through, the final stage is for the burn reconstruction team and the patient to agree a plan of action. This may be simple and involve one minor procedure, or highly complex involving staged procedures over a considerable period of time.

Timing

Most reconstruction will be delayed until scars have fully matured (~2 years) and effects of scar management have declared themselves, unless early intervention is warranted due to severe functional impediment or deformity. Correct surgical timing is pivotal: operating too early may worsen eventual outcome. As children are growing, the timing of surgical interventions is particularly important, too early and it might be necessary to repeat a procedure, too late and there might be permanent effects on movement due to secondary joint tightness.

Further reading

Brou JA, Robson MC, McCauley RL, et al. Inventory of potential reconstructive needs in the patient with burns. Journal of Burn Care and Rehabilitation 1989;10:555–60.

Donelan MB. Principles of burn reconstruction. In Thorne CH (ed.) Grabb and Smith's plastic surgery, 6th edn. Philadelphia: Lippincott, 2007.

Shokrollahi K, Whitaker IS, Nahai F (eds). Flaps: practical reconstructive surgery. Stuttgart: Thieme 2017.

Wainwright DJ. Burn reconstruction: the problems, the techniques and the applications. Clinics in Plastic Surgery 2009;36:687–700.

Burn contracture surgery

Prevention of contractures

Many burn scar problems can be prevented by appropriate intervention and work from the burns multidisciplinary team (which includes the patient). Typical interventions include the following.

Nurses
- Prevention of infection
- Encourage mobilization

Surgeons
- Skin grafting to achieve early healing

Patient and family
- Compliance with exercises, massage, splints, and pressure garments

Physiotherapist/occupational therapist
- Crucial role in encouraging and providing physical rehabilitation; instilling determination and compliance with rehabilitation regime in the patient and family
- Manufacture and fitting of splints, moulds, silicone, and pressure garments for scar therapy

Anaesthesia/pain management
- Providing physical comfort so that patient can mobilize stiff joints

Contracture definitions

Intrinsic contracture
A contracture where scarring directly involves the site affected by contraction.

Extrinsic contracture
A contracture of normal structures that are pulled out of position by scarring distant to the site. A typical example of this is a normal lower eyelid pulled into ectropion by scarring on the cheek.

Linear band contracture
A band of scar tissue surrounded by relatively normal skin. This is readily treatable by local flap plasties with or without band excision.

Linear band contracture in diffuse scarring
The skin surrounding a band contracture is scarred and Z plasties that require flap elevation carry a high risk of necrosis. Y–V plasties that do not require flap elevation may be an option. However, in scarred skin, the Y–V plasties may simply move the site of the troublesome band to an adjacent area, and a larger flap or graft may be required instead.

Broadband contracture
The contracture involves the whole of an anatomical surface and requires an incisional release or excision with inset of flap or graft to make good the skin deficit.

Joint contracture
In addition to the skin contracture, ligaments, muscles, and tendons have shortened or ruptured to cause a secondary joint deformity that requires treatment.

Timing of contracture surgery: indications

Urgent
- Upper eyelid retraction causing exposure of cornea
- Severe neck contracture
- Severe oral contracture

Early
During period when scars are most active; arbitrarily in the first 6 months:
- Lower eyelid contracture causing ectropion, infection, discomfort
- Oral contracture
- Neck contracture
- Upper limb contracture interfering with important functions
- Lower limb contractures impairing ambulation
- Unstable scar with infection/osteomyelitis
  - Osteomyelitis must be treated *per se* before soft tissue cover is attempted

Late
- Contractures persisting after scar therapy and resolution
- Troublesome persistent hypertrophic scars, especially unstable scars
- Any contracture treated for aesthetic reasons
  - as a general rule, one should wait about 2 years minimum to allow scars to resolve as far as possible before operating for reasons of appearance

General principles and technical tips

- Identify and mark the contracture pre-operatively. It is important to assess the position and posture in which the contracture is tightest pre-operatively
- Try to diagnose underlying joint contracture preoperatively
- Remember that a contracture has arisen because of a **deficit of skin**, and that surgery should de designed to replace that deficit. Often it is a fascinating challenge to decide whether this can be done with local skin or whether additional skin needs to be imported
- Ascertain whether the contracture is predominantly a linear band, which might be amenable to a local flap procedure or whether it is a broadband contracture, which requires additional skin in the form of a graft or larger flap. If a linear contracture is also surrounded by scarred skin, deciding on the best technique may be more challenging. In such cases, err towards putting in more skin via flap or graft rather than using local flap plasties which tend to be associated with persistent contracture
- In children, do not be tempted to 'cheat' and use a local flap plasty type procedure when additional skin is needed in a linear contracture with diffuse scar or a broadband contracture. Even if a release can be achieved, as the patient grows, the scar tightness will soon recur
- Use full thickness grafts or flaps when reasonably possible rather than split skin grafts or dermal substitutes. Split skin grafts and dermal substitutes shrink during healing and require more aftercare (splints, pressure garments and physiotherapy) than do full thickness grafts or flaps. However, note that often a spilt thickness graft or dermal substitute plus graft are the only realistic options for extensive contractures
- When a person has survived an extensive deep burn injury, choose your donor sites carefully: there may be a precious donor site which is crucial for a future reconstruction that you should avoid using for an earlier procedure (eg. if a patient may need facial resurfacing later, keep a good donor site for large sheet grafts)
- It is very important to release all subcutaneous scar bands as well as the cutaneous bands
- When incising to release a contracture, it is tempting to simply cut deeper and deeper in the initial line of release. Once incision has passed through the full thickness of the subcutaneous scar, incision in the centre of the defect should cease, and incision recommences at the proximal and distal margins of the initial skin incision
- After an extensive incisional release it is often best to excise some of the scarred skin edges otherwise skin edge necrosis is likely to compromise healing

Important rule: Keep incising at the margins of the defect. Don't keep going deep in the centre once you are through all the depth of the contraction scar.

- When skin grafting, excise as much of the subcutaneous scar as possible to achieve a well-vascularized bed for your graft. Scar is a very poor bed for a skin graft. If your graft fails, the contracture will almost certainly recur. This is especially important for dermal substitutes that require a scar free bed for consistent take
- When creating a release prior to skin grafting, create the largest defect reasonably possible so that as much extra tissue is inserted as possible. When a flap of normal skin is used to repair the defect, a slightly less extensive release may be effective, as the flap can stretch with time
- If you are incising to release a contracture and it is not releasing as well as you hope, **excise** some of the scar. Often this will enhance the release
- Commonly after a scar release, the defect for skin grafting will be deeply concave. Use a good-sized graft that contours well into the defect, and a tie-over dressing to control the graft. If the bed is very irregularly contoured, mesh the graft to improve take (eg. axilla)

Topical negative pressure dressings are a good alternative to tie-over dressings and have been shown to be particularly useful with dermal substitutes.

- In the upper limb, release contractures proximal to distal (eg. shoulder–elbow–hand or wrist–palm–fingers). This may have to be done in staged operations, or can be done in a single procedure
- Operating on the hand: document sensation preoperatively and don't cut the digital nerves
- If a patient has multiple contractures, it is often advantageous to operate on several contractures in the same procedure
- Try to avoid excessive distress (especially postoperative pain) for the patient. He/she may need many operations

Approach to contracture surgery

Plan carefully: involve the patient and therapist in the decision-making process as much as possible. Often the choice of technique for treating a contracture will be influenced by the patient's own views and preferences for donor tissue. Try to have a holistic approach that takes account of the patient's current and future needs from a physical, social, and psychological point of view. It may be useful to involve the team psychologist in the planning process.

Make sure the patient understands that a graft or flap is likely to look like a 'patch' and may look especially bad early or after the surgery. Warn about scar hypertrophy and aftercare.

Get to know the patient and counsel him/her carefully before doing anything major from a surgical point of view. Sometimes it is useful to start off with quite a minor surgical procedure if possible so that the patient understands that surgery is not necessarily an aversive experience (primary burn treatment is likely to bring unpleasant memories).

Have a number of 'workhorse' procedures, which you use for different types of contracture, and get to know these techniques.

For example:

- We tend to use Y–V plasties for long linear bands, except in the neck where we use Zs because a Z puts some of the scar in a transverse crease. We use Zs or five-flap plasties for short bands
- We use a lot of full thickness grafts for broadband contractures. Commonly these grafts are harvested by abdominoplasty or mini-abdominoplasty
- Around the axilla, we use a lot of local flaps because there is often skin laxity with many perforators and the circumflex scapular and thoracodorsal vessels
- We use a two-stage dermal substitute for resurfacing and for extensive contractures
- We use free flaps for difficult contractures

The aforementioned are not necessarily the 'best' techniques for every indication, but there is a great advantage to surgeon and patient in using a technique that is familiar and has the highest chance of working. Different surgeons will have their own techniques that are most reliable in their hands.

An ambitious and elegant technique that fails can be a disaster for the patient.

Split skin grafts

For the most extensive and severe contractures, split skin graft is often the only technique that will supply sufficient extra skin to make good the massive deficit. If a large thick split skin graft is required (eg. for severe neck or hand contracture), consider overgrafting the donor site for this skin graft with a much thinner adjacent graft, so as to avoid problem of severe delay in donor site healing. (However, it is important to warn the patient that the overgrafted donor site leaves a scar which may be aesthetically unsatisfactory.)

Thin split skin grafts tend to shrink postoperatively and have a high incidence of recurrence of contracture. Their use is not recommendation for burn reconstruction.

Full thickness grafts

Full thickness grafts are extremely useful for moderate-sized defects after incisional release of contracture or scar excision. The abdomen is the typical donor site via various transverse lower abdominal incisions including abdominoplasty. Postauricular and supraclavicular can provide the colour match desired for facial skin (the latter can be pre-expanded to resurface larger facial defects). Any other site of skin laxity permitting direct closure may be used included various innovative options (eg. skin harvest from the undersurface of breast via a reduction or mastopexy).

Grafts tend to be 'large' in comparison to the average full thickness graft for other indications, so the graft should be thinned carefully to remove fat from the deep surface, and great care taken to remove all scar from the recipient bed so as to encourage good take.

Careful compressive dressings such as tie-over or tie through dressings are generally used, and splints used on the limbs.

Full thickness grafts generally require less aftercare than most grafts, although if there is patchy take, scar hypertrophy and pigmentation problems may occur, so the patient should be warned of these potential occurrences and possible treatments.

Dermal substitutes

Dermal substitutes (also known as dermal regeneration template or matrix) are very useful for burn contractures, especially in patients with a paucity of good donor sites. Thin skin autografts are used with the dermal substitute to produce an outcome that varies in quality from that achieved with a thin/medium/thick split skin graft, depending how well the dermal component has taken. In most cases, the result does not achieve the quality of a full thickness graft (or normal skin), and aftercare with pressure garments and splints is typically required for dermal substitutes.

They are indicated for broadband contractures and for resurfacing of extensive areas after scar excision.

Use of dermal substitutes is more demanding technically than split autografts, with higher risk of infection. It is critically important to excise all of the scar from the bed to achieve good take, and in the neck it is considered best to excise platysma from the bed for good take of dermal substitute.

Two-stage dermal substitute is a collagneous matrix that has a silicone external layer: the external layer remains in situ for 2–3 weeks before secondary thin autograft is applied.

One-stage dermal collagen matrices may have the autograft applied at time of application.

Key technical points

- Completely release the contracture so there is no residual tension or distortion
- Use tie-over dressings or topical negative pressure dressings plus splints where indicated: shearing is a disaster for these grafts
- Be very careful about infection; prophylactic antibiotics are commonly indicated
- Avoid excessive frequency of dressing changes
- Single stage may look very 'tatty' in early weeks, but still re-epithelialize well
- Have a good aftercare programme

Local flaps

Where suitable tissue exists, a local flap procedure, either by some type of 'plasty' or by a flap transfer such as an islanded ad hoc perforator flap, is close to the ideal method of contracture release, providing reliability, good tissue colour match, and little need for aftercare. However, the temptation always exists for the surgeon to 'force' a technique to treat a contracture when there is insufficient tissue available, with a variety of adverse consequences.

Even where tissue is available poor outcomes may result from undue bulk of many specific locoregional flaps (eg. unthinned scapular flaps for the axilla) so careful assessment and good judgement are pre-requisites for application of local flap techniques.

Free flaps

Free flaps may be very useful for difficult contractures and complex defects especially in the head and neck, and the upper and lower limbs. Commonly recipient vessels are undamaged by the burn injury (except in electrical injuries where more caution is necessary).

The greatest challenge is often to match the contour and colour (some flaps tend to be too bulky and normal skin may look aesthetically incongruous in the centre of an area of scar).

A multiplicity of different options is available, and discussion of these is beyond the scope of this chapter. However, our experience is that burn patients tend to do well with free tissue transfer when well counselled and prepared. It is commonly possible to use the relatively long anaesthetic to address several other contractures at the same time.

Tissue expansion

Tissue expansion tends to be of particular value for treatment of severe scars causing aesthetic embarrassment. Examples include post-burn alopecia and partial facial or neck defects in which there is normal skin available to expand in order to resurface a scarred area with local tissue of appropriate colour, texture, and hair growth.

Patient counselling is of great importance. Incisions should be placed radial to the expander where possible to reduce the likelihood of dehiscence and exposure.

Flaps should be 'over-expanded' as almost always there is more retraction of expanded skin than one expects. Where possible, incisions for flaps in hairless skin should follow aesthetic unit principles.

Techniques used in different anatomical sites: important note

The following sections deal with different anatomical areas in three regions: the upper limb, the head and neck, and the groin/perineum and lower limb regions.

For relative brevity, various methods have only been illustrated in one or two anatomical sites (eg. perforator-based propeller flap is illustrated for antecubital fossa, but it can readily be applied in many different sites such as axilla, groin, popliteal fossa, and leg/foot). Square flaps and asymmetric Z plasties can be used in many sites.

Many of the techniques are applicable to many different sites. To some extent the selection of techniques illustrated represents the author's own experience and bias, but ultimately the choice of technique is determined by many factors that include the following:

- The nature of the contracture
- Necessity for surgery on underlying joint (more likely to need flap)
- Availability of local tissue
- Availability of good graft donor sites
- Age of patient (more likely to use graft/dermal regeneration template in child)
- Compliance of patient (more likely to use flap or free flap in less well compliant patient who will not do aftercare)
- Wishes of the patient (eg. are they keen to have an abdominoplasty that might allow harvest of a big full thickness graft?)
- How long can patient take off work/childcare/school/university etc.?
- Any problem with infections? (less likely to use dermal template or tissue expansion)

The upper limb

The hand

General principles

Generally, aim to release significant contractures of axilla and antecubital fossa before operating on the hand. Technically, it is very difficult to operate on the hand with the major proximal joints contracted. Functionally, the hand is severely impaired if the limb is adducted at shoulder and flexed at elbow.

Release from proximal to distal in the hand itself: release of the proximal wrist/palm contracture makes it much easier to operate on the digits.

Operate with tourniquet to produce a bloodless field. Do not keep tourniquet inflated for >2 hours to minimize risk of ischaemia or nerve palsy. As a general principle, following contracture release, deflate tourniquet and apply compressive gauze dressing, prior to taking graft so that haemostasis in complete by time graft is applied.

Use bipolar diathermy and magnifying glasses.

Always have regard for the anatomy of the digital nerves and vessels.

Local flap 'plasties' in the hand

Underlying principles

- Local flap plasties are most useful for relatively narrow contraction bands
- Avoid damage to digital nerves, but raise flaps as thick as possible to protect vascularity of flap
- Effectiveness of release with local flap plasties depends on there being reasonable soft tissue laxity in a transverse plane
- In children who have a significant amount of scarring, release with local flaps in the hand may be short-lived (with effect of growth) and full thickness grafts may be a better option to produce a long-term benefit

Five-flap Z plasty

This is made up of two Z plasties and a central Y–V plasty.

This technique is particularly useful for moderate contractures of the first web where there is laxity of tissue at 90° to the direction of the contraction band (Fig. 30.1).

It is also occasionally useful for moderate contractures of the flexor surface of the digits.

Z plasty

Multiple Zs are good on the flexor surface of the fingers for linear contraction bands (more often after trauma than burns) Angle of Zs is usually 60°.

A single large Z is excellent for deepening the first web when there is relatively little scarring or a very tight but narrow contraction band.

With moderate or severe diffuse scarring, there is a high risk of Z-plasty flap necrosis, because of requirement to undermine flaps to allow transposition.

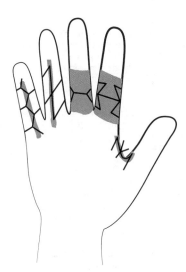

Fig. 30.1 Diagram showing possible design of local flap procedures for linear band contractures on little, ring finger and first web. For more severe diffuse contractures shown on the index and middle fingers, the methods of incisional release with either lateral Z plasties (double trapezoid flaps) or fishtail darts are shown reaching midlateral lines. These more severe contractures ideally require full thickness skin grafts, or possibly thick split thickness grafts.

Y–V plasty

This is an excellent technique for linear contraction bands in moderately scarred skin. Because the flaps of a Y–V plasty do not have to be undermined, there is less risk of skin flap tip necrosis. Conversely, a greater length of incision is required than with a Z plasty, hence the 'Z' is more elegant where there is less diffuse scarring.

Skin grafting and flaps for hand contractures

Palmar surface—flexion contractures

Where possible, full thickness grafts should be used on the flexor surface of the hand. Other options include split skin grafts from the instep (no weight-bearing) surface of the sole of foot, or thick split skin grafts.

For severe palm contractures, excision of a central portion of the scar with extensive incisional release usually produces a bed that is graftable. When grafting, it is important to excise as much of the scar from the bed as possible, so that a well-vascularized surface is produced. K wiring of the digits in extension for several weeks is usually essential to optimize the outcome.

Important technical points
- Surgery should be undertaken under tourniquet
- Release proximal contractures (wrist/palm) before the fingers
- On the digits, it is important to design the release so that grafts reach the mid-lateral line on each side of the finger. This prevents the scar at the margin of the graft from re-contracting
- The margins of the grafts should be zig-zagged or the release. planned with lateral Zs—the trapezoid flap) (see the index finger in Fig 30.1)
- Great care should be taken to avoid damage to the digital nerves and arteries. These can easily be mistaken for scar bands. Operating using magnification is essential
- On extension of the digit in a severe contracture, ischaemia may result—usually this is transient and relates to tethering of the digital vessels. Either reducing the degree of extension or (preferred) extending the release of scarring, will allow the flow to recover (as long as the digital arteries have not been divided!)

In severe palmar contractures after very deep burns, it is sometimes necessary to use a flap if burn extends through palmar fascia (eg. electrical injury). One of the simplest options is a radial forearm fascial flap covered by a skin graft. This avoids excessive bulk. Alternatives are a well-thinned pedicled groin flap or a Becker flap. The latter has the advantage of being a single-stage transfer, although both the groin flap and Becker flap are almost certain to require secondary thinning if used for a palm defect.

A variety of thin free flap options may be used, such as free fascial flaps, radically thinned free muscle flaps (covered by graft), or perforator based free thin skin flaps.

After such very deep injuries assessment needs to be made as to whether reconstruction of digitals nerves or flexor tendons is indicated and/or feasible. A useful passive range of joint movement and good resting posture of the hand are essential prior to undertaking such complex reconstructions.

The PIPJ flexion deformity

Often, release of the proximal interphalangeal joint (PIPJ) is difficult in established contractures because of contracture of the volar plate and accessory collateral ligaments. In children, it is possible to stretch these by strong steady pressure, but care should be exercised to avoid overstretching the digital nerves and arteries. In older patients, with a long history, release of the volar plate and accessory collaterals may be indicated. Where possible, this should be carried out through a lateral approach around the side of the neurovascular bundles so as to avoid exposing flexor tendon through the defect to be skin grafted. The joint should be K wired in extension postoperatively. If the flexor sheath is opened, a skin graft will often 'bridge' across a small defect which exposes flexor tendon, especially if the finger is kept extended with a K wire.

Extensor surface—extension contractures

Skin grafting

These contractures are common and usually respond well to excision of a small portion of the scar and extensive incisional release with medium thickness split skin graft. Ideally, this should be carried out superficial to the large veins of the dorsum of the hand, producing an excellent bed for the graft to take, and allow tendon gliding. However, in deeper burn injuries, release may have to be undertaken superficial to the extensor paratenon.

Commonly the metacarpophalangeal joints (MCPJs) are contracted in an extended position and a dorsal MCPJ capsulotomy is required. Usually this is done through a separate longitudinal incision to avoid exposing the joint in the release. K wiring or splinting the MCPJs in flexion postoperatively for several weeks is essential to maintaining the correction.

Occasionally, extensive hypertrophic scarring of the dorsum of the hand may be resurfaced with thick skin graft or dermal substitute. Meticulous aftercare is required.

Severe dorsal contractures (role of flaps)

Commonly, more severe dorsal contractures involve the extensors tendons, or are associated with severe hyperextension/subluxation of the MCPJ and IPJ flexion. To achieve a release, the tendons and possibly MCPJ will have to be exposed without paratenon cover. A flap is commonly required, and the fingers may need to be temporarily syndactylized up to PIPJ. MCPJ capsulotomy and K wiring of MCPJs in flexion in required. PIPJ release is often necessary with palmar skin grafting and K wiring.

Useful flaps in this situation are a reverse radial forearm flap (although it cannot readily reach distal to mid-proximal phalanx level if covering the whole width of the dorsum) or a free flap (thin tissue should be used if possible).

A pedicled groin flap is a very safe alternative, but is associated with significant stiffness and oedema and almost always requires secondary thinning. If the hand is very scarred the groin flap has to be left attached for longer than usual as vascularization through scarred skin is poor (3 weeks rather than 2).

For smaller, more proximal defects on the dorsum of the hand, a Becker flap may be used.

Interdigital web contractures

Mild dorsal or palmar web contractures can readily be released by 5-flap Z plasty or by the square flap technique (Fig. 30.2)

If scarring is more severe, incision and full thickness grafting is required. Often the defect to be grafted is quite concave, and a tie-over dressing is required. A rectangular dorsal flap as in congenital syndactyly can help to create a web in severe contractures, with the defects on the sides of the fingers, repaired with full thickness grafts.

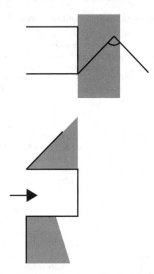

Fig. 30.2 Square flap technique that can be used for linear band contractures of moderate thickness and provides optimal geometric lengthening. The square flap in healthy skin advances into flaps of same side length in the contracture band with angles of 45° and 90°. This technique is unlikely to work at all well if the skin is heavily scarred around the square flap.

The axilla

Adduction contracture of the axilla is very common after burn injury. A variety of options are available.

Procedures for linear band contractures

The type of discrete linear band contracture shown could readily be released with multiple Y–V plasties or multiple Z plasties. Our preferred option is Y–V because of minimal risk of skin flap tip necrosis (the flaps do not have to be undermined).

The Y–Vs should be continued for the length of the contraction band to provide a good release. All subcutaneous scar should be incised. The stems of the Ys should be as long as reasonable tension permits to allow optimum advancement of the flaps. The interdigitating flaps break up and lengthen the contracture (see Fig. 30.3).

Perforator-based flaps for axilla

A wealth of perforator-based flaps are available around the axilla They may be raised on known vessels, or as 'ad hoc' perforator flaps based on vessels near the defect using a 'propeller' design. Figs 30.3 and 30.4 show two flaps which we have found to be consistently reliable. We find it helpful to use magnifying glasses so as to visualise the perforating vessels in the flap base.

Medial Arm Flap for Thick anterior axilla/shoulder band

The medial arm flap is centred approximately over the line of the medial intermuscular septum of the arm. It is based on perforators which emerge from the axilla, and on the medial cutaneous nerve of the arm (it is not to

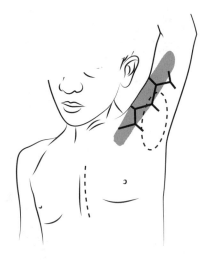

Fig. 30.3 Multiple Y–V for axillary band.

be confused with the classical medial arm free flap, whose pedicle emerges more distally) (Fig. 30.4).

Posterior arm flap

This is a similar flap to the medial arm fasciocutaneous flap. This flap is based on a perforating artery, which arises from the axilla at the base of the posterior axillary fold. The flap is widely used for repair of axillary hair bearing skin after excision for infection (hidradenitis suppurativa). It is occasionally useful for burn contractures where the posterior fold area is spared and the posterior arm relatively scar-free (see Fig. 30.5).

Procedures for diffuse axillary contractures

Flaps

For a broadband axillary contracture, a variety of flaps are available. Note that application of any of these flaps depends on whether sufficient healthy skin is available to allow design of a flap, which can be transposed to cover the axilla. This is commonly not the case.

Flaps require less splintage and aftercare than grafts, although they not uncommonly require secondary thinning.

The simplest flaps are fasciocutaneous and perforator-based flaps that are based on the axilla or adjacent area, and involve harvest of a flap of skin from the arm (see above, medial arm, posterior arm) or from the chest wall below the axilla. Propeller flaps and the islanded perforator-based

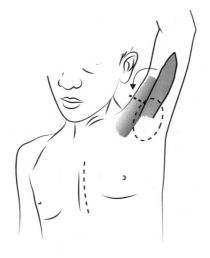

Fig. 30.4 This medial arm flap is a fasciocutaneous flap based in the axilla and harvested from the medial aspect of the arm. It is designed at a width that allows primary closure of the donor defect. The medial cutaneous nerve of the arm is included in the flap. The flap is transposed 90° and is inset into defect after release of a broadband anterior axillary fold contracture.

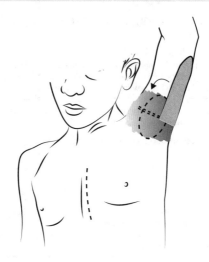

Fig 30.5 Posterior arm flap based on perforating vessel in posterior axillary fold.

development of propeller flaps have been widely used for axillary contractures of moderate severity.

More complex flaps used for the axilla include the scapular, parascapular and latissimus dorsi. these may occasionally be indicated for very severe contractures requiring a very deep release, but are generally somewhat bulky, and are relatively complex to raise (the scapular flaps in particular are tricky to raise for the less experienced surgeon).

Grafting
Split skin grafting is often necessary in severe axillary contractures where no local tissue is available to design a flap. The defect for grafting is often deeply concave; so a tie-over dressing is essential, and a 1:1.5 meshed graft is often helpful to achieving good graft take. In severe contractures, release of some fibres of the pectoralis major is occasionally required to help with the release. An abduction splint is used for 2–3 weeks and physiotherapy exercises are essential thereafter to prevent graft shrinkage.

Trapezoid flap plus grafting
A trapezoid flap is an excellent method of releasing a broadband axillary contracture with diffuse scarring.

The principle is to use the flap to move stable scarred skin up into the axilla from the lateral chest wall below the axilla and to place the graft on the resultant defect on the lateral chest wall (a more favourable site for graft take than the concave, irregular axilla). Because the graft is not directly over the joint, more rapid mobilization of the shoulder may be undertaken (Fig. 30.6).

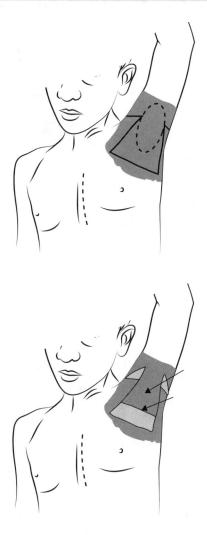

Fig. 30.6 (A) Flap advancing to axilla. (B) Keep incising at this edge, not undermining. (C) Flap is advanced to axilla and Zs at margins of flap are close. Defect for skin graft created by release.

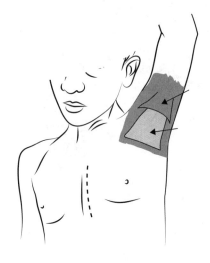

Fig. 30.6 (Contd.)

Antecubital fossa

Local flaps for mild/moderate scarring

A variety of local flap procedures are useful for linear contractures of the antecubital fossa.

In long linear band contractures involving both the axilla and antecubital fossa, multiple Y–V plasties offer a simple solution, albeit one which leaves a long incision and significant scarring.

For moderately thick linear band contractures, an asymmetric Z plasty may provide a useful release without excessive additional scarring, as long as there is skin laxity and adjacent normal skin for the Z flaps to be elevated (see Fig. 30.7).

Propeller flap or island perforator-based flap

The 'propeller' principle has been applied using a single island flap based on a perforating vessel. The flap may be rotated by as much as 180°. There tends to be many perforating vessels close to the elbow joint, and hence a flap can be planned and transposed into a defect after release of a moderately broad contracture.

Increasingly, such flaps are being termed 'propeller' flaps. Alternative descriptive terms for the propeller flap are island perforator flap or ad hoc perforator flap (Fig. 30.8).

Diffuse contractures of antecubital fossa

For diffuse contractures, incisional release and skin grafting is reliable. The 'fishtail' design is commonly used, care being taken to release to the mid lateral lines. A good alternative is to use an incisional release with Z plasties at each margin.

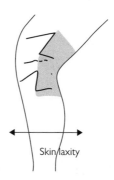

Skin laxity

Fig. 30.7 Asymmetric Z plasty. The 90° limbs of the flaps are placed in the scar and should be incised through full thickness of scar but not undermined. The 60° flaps in healthy skin are undermined.

Sometimes incisional release at the elbow crease tends to carry dissection deep, requiring division of the cephalic vein and reaching close to the brachial artery and median nerve which lie relatively superficial at the line of the elbow.

A technique which avoids the problem of excessively deep release at the line of the elbow crease is to use two incisions, proximal and distal to the elbow crease line, about 6 cm apart, so that a patch of skin is preserved over the antecubital fossa and grafts are inserted proximal and distal to this. This allows an effective contracture release without excessively deep dissection (Fig.30.9).

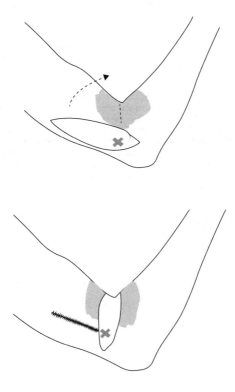

Fig. 30.8 (A) Island or ad hoc perforator flap. Perforator in base of flap. (B) Islanded and transposed.

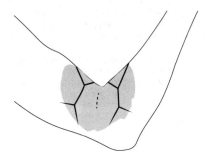

Fig. 30.9 Double incisional release at elbow. This leaves skin intact over median nerve and brachial artery and allows the skin grafts to be inset to good beds over the brachial and forearm muscles.

For severe contractures of the antecubital fossa, a very extensive release may be required, and sometimes this may include release biceps tendon and some fibres of brachialis. In this event, larger flaps are required at the antecubutal fossa. The indication for this is a release, which extends down to brachial artery and median nerve, and/or a tendon lengthening procedure. If a flap is essential, a proximally based radial forearm flap, or a distally based medial or lateral arm flap may be used. Almost always, the donor defect for these flaps has to be skin grafted. A free flap may be a good option for such severe cases.

The olecranon

Quite commonly, the olecranon becomes exposed after flame burn injury of the upper limb. While not strictly speaking a contracture, this is often a problem for the patient, with persistent scar breakdown and discomfort.

Often, this will gradually heal with time, so it is worth persisting with dressings and topical and systemic antibiotics.

If the area persistently fails to heal, a variety local transposition or advancement flaps may be used, depending on where there is local skin laxity (skin free of scarring).

If there is no local skin laxity, a distally based lateral arm fascial flap or a proximally based posterior interosseous flap may be used to provide thin tissue to cover the olecranon.

The wrist

Flexion contracture of the wrist is a common consequence of flame burn injury or electrical burn.

After burns of moderate depth, release and medium thickness split skin graft or full thickness graft will commonly produce a satisfactory result.

The wrist should be splinted in extension for several weeks afterwards and at night for several months.

Occasionally, in more severe contractures it is helpful to sacrifice the flexor carpi radialis tendon, preserving the fascia over the deeper flexor tendons. (The palmaris longus can always be sacrificed.)

After very deep burns, such as an electrical burn, release may expose tendons and median nerve (which may be damaged and may even require reconstruction). In this event, a flap is required to cover the flexor aspect of the wrist.

Free flaps offer most flexible coverage and tissue components for these complex defects with the possibility of bi-layered flaps of skin and fascia to wrap tendons or nerve grafts, and various other composite tissue options.

The pedicled groin flap is a reliable option for these defects. Occasionally, the much simpler Becker flap may be transposed (distally based) from the ulnar aspect of the forearm to cover the flexor aspect of the wrist if the perforating vessel from the ulnar artery is intact.

For linear band contractures of the wrist, Y–V plasties or multiple Z plasties are suitable.

Head and neck

Neck contractures

Linear band contractures—Z plasty

Discrete neck contraction bands can be very effectively treated with Z plasties. Depending on the length of the band, either a large single or multiple Zs can be used. We have found these give superior aesthetic results to Y–V plasties in the neck, probably because the transverse limb of the Z lies in a line of election.

Technical points

- Mark the contracture band preoperatively
- Position the patient with a roll under shoulders to extend the neck
- Raise the flaps with a good thickness of subcutaneous fat to avoid tip necrosis
- Release all subcutaneous bands
- Take care to avoid the external jugular vein laterally and the especially accessory nerve further laterally
- Use 1 in 200,000 adrenaline solution to reduce intraoperative bleeding. It is useful to include local anaesthetic in the solution for postoperative pain relief (Fig. 30.10)

Diffuse (broadband) neck contractures

Diffuse neck contractures are a common complication of upper body flame burns. They commonly require surgery early after injury because of difficulties with function and especially with protecting the airway for anaesthesia.

Typically, thick split thickness or full thickness grafts are used for resurfacing after release of broad neck contractures. Generally, it is considered best to carry the releasing incision through platysma and to excise the platysma in the base of the release. Dermal template may also be used for grafting if insufficient autograft is available (Figs 30.11 and 30.12).

Technical points

- Excision of a little of the scar on either side of the incision helps with achieving a wide release and prevents marginal skin necrosis at the edge of the release.
- It is of the utmost importance to carry the release far laterally. So as to avoid lateral persistence of contracture.
- A trapezoid or double trapezoid flap (Fig. 30.12) is a useful method of release of neck contractures, especially for contractures that are wide but do not extend the full width of the neck. The Z plasties at the margins help to prevent marginal contracture.
- Occasionally, bleeding may be severe. Adrenaline infiltration is helpful, and care should be taken to avoid excessive haemorrhage.
- A rare, but potentially devastating complication is of air embolism via the external jugular vein. If the vein is opened inadvertently, the vein should be compressed and the patient should be placed head down for repair or clamping of the vein. (Also applies to internal jugular which may rarely be encountered in a contracture.)

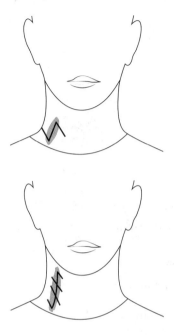

Fig. 30.10 Diagram showing possible design of Z plasties for neck contractures. The typical angle of the oblique limb to the vertical limb of the z plasties should be 60°, but this can be varied. Excessively acute angles (<45° may lead to skin flap necrosis).

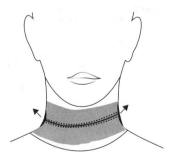

Fig. 30.11 Release carried laterally.

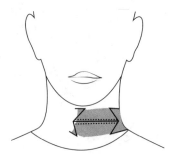

Fig. 30.12 Double trapezoid flaps.

- Great care should be taken in releasing scars in the line between the ear lobule and acromion, to avoid the accessory nerve.
- A concave defect results from release. Skin grafts should be secured with a tie over (or similar) dressing. Negative pressure dressings are also useful for securing grafts or dermal substitutes. There is a small risk of postoperative external respiratory obstruction from haemorrhage/compression under the tie-over dressing. Staff looking after the patient should be warned to remove the tie-over immediately if stridor and respiratory distress are present.

Flaps for neck contractures

Free flaps may be very useful for neck contractures, but the surgery is relatively demanding. Consistent recipient vessels are the superior thyroid artery and the internal and external jugular veins.

It can be particularly challenging to obtain free flap tissue that does not have excessive bulk. Options include 'thin' perforator flaps, such as anterolateral thigh flaps; a radial or ulnar forearm flap (poorer donor site); pre-expanded flaps (much more complex for patient). The big advantage of a free flap is minimum requirement for aftercare and corresponding immediate benefit for these uncomfortable contractures.

It is important to put transverse/lateral tension on the flap to pull it into the contour of the neck. However if this risks compromising vascularity by pressure on the pedicle, this can be left for a second stage.

In thin patients, a latissimus dorsi or thoracodorsal artery perforator flap may be used for a neck contracture.

The face

The eyelids

Generally burn contractures of the eyelids are released with grafts. Z plasties are very useful after trauma or congenital problems, but uncommonly in burns.

Upper eyelid

Retraction of the upper eyelid requires urgent release with a skin graft. If possible the graft should be inserted about 9–10 mm above the lid margin in a curve which lies in the line of the normal upper lid crease (This may not always be possible if the lid has retracted very high, or if there is severe pretarsal burn). The scar is released superficial to orbicularis, creating as large a defect for a graft as reasonably possible and extending medially and laterally to the orbital margins.

Occasionally, in a very deep burn, the graft may have to be placed on orbital septum.

Conventionally, medium to thick split skin grafts have been used for the upper eyelid, both so as to preserve the best donor sites for full thickness grafts for later reconstruction around the face, and because full thickness grafts tend to be stiff when used in the upper eyelid.

Lower eyelid

Typically lower eyelid contractures (causing ectropion) are released with full thickness skin grafts from the post-auricular area or supraclavicular fossa that give the best colour match for facial skin.

The release can be carried out in a 'melon-slice' shape, or be extended more laterally towards the temple, reaching the orbital margin. Both methods tend to give a good correction, although the latter tends to give a superior aesthetic result. Generally, the bigger the graft, the better the aesthetic result because of avoidance of scars on the lid itself.

Upper and lower eyelid contractures—technical points

- Infiltrate with 1 in 200000 Adrenaline solution with a fine hypodermic needle to reduce bleeding. Use bipolar diathermy as precisely as possible to avoid necrotic patches under the grafts
- Try to create as large a defect as reasonably possible to make an optimum release
- After upper eyelid release, insert a temporary tarsorraphy suture between the centre of the lids to splint the upper eyelid in position
- After lower eyelid release, a suture can be placed in the centre of the lower eyelid and taped up to the forehead to splint the lid in position (Frost suture)
- Use tie-over dressings. It helps if the 'bolus' for the tie-over is stiff and matches the contour of the lid to avoid the tie over pulling the conjunctiva and tarsus away from the eye. Options include using K wire around the edge of bolus dressings or making a bolus of thermoplastic mouldable plastic splint to fashion a semi rigid bolus for tie over dressing
- Use antibiotic eye ointment to prevent infection and desiccation

Occasionally, lower eyelid contractures are caused by severe scarring of the cheek rather than by intrinsic contracture of the lid itself (extrinsic contracture). In this event, release should ideally include some form of release or resurfacing of the cheek scar too, to avoid an incomplete release.

The mouth

Early on after facial burn injury, microstomia may result from severe scar contracture. To a degree this can be prevented by frequent use of oral splints, but there are often problems with patient compliance.

Commonly it is necessary to release the oral commissures early after burn injury if increasing tightness occurs. Our preferred method is to do a Y–V plasty where a V-shaped flap of oral mucosa is planned on the inside of the mouth with the apex of the V at the commissure. The V is made into a Y with an external transverse incision from the commissure running laterally for about 1 cm. The V flap is incised and the stem of the Y is incised to divide the contracted commissure. Often some orbicularis muscle has to be divided. It is a difficult judgement to know how much of this to divide as it is an important muscle for oral continence, so it is best to err on the side of caution if in doubt. The V flap is then advanced into the transverse external defect. Often small 'Burow' triangles of vermillion or oral mucosa have to be trimmed above and below the inset flap to allow it to inset neatly.

This minor procedure often has to be repeated after a few months on a couple of occasions, but this seems preferable in the long term to very unsightly rectangular patches of skin graft inset at each commissure, which is the typical alternative to release commissure scars.

Severe scarring often restricts movement of upper and lower lips and causes retraction of upper lip and ectropion of the lower lip with various functional problems. However, unless this is very severe, it is best to give these scars time to mature before undertaking revision (1–2 years)

Where possible, the lips should be released and the upper lip skin and chin resurfaced with good sized 'aesthetic unit' grafts rather than attempting piecemeal releases with Zs or small grafts.

Using large grafts on the aesthetic unit principle generally gives much better functional and aesthetic results, than attempting minimum sized grafts.

If resurfacing the face for aesthetic reasons, wait till scar resolution is well advanced, and stick to aesthetic unit principles for resurfacing facial scars.

An occasional exception to this is when isolated raised hypertrophic scars can be shaved down, grafted and treated with pressure to improve overt lumpiness. This requires careful aftercare.

Anaesthesia

For face and neck contracture surgery it is essential to involve the anaesthetist in the decision-making process as there are many ways in which the airway can be compromised at induction of anaesthesia, during and after surgery.

Groin/perineum and lower limb

Groin and perineum

Flexion contractures of the hip result from tight scars across the anterior aspect of the inguinal are and thigh.

For Linear band contractures, Z plasty, Y–V plasty, or local transposition/propeller flaps may be used depending on the dimensions of the band (Figs 30.13 and 30.14).

Rarely a contracture in this area may need a flap (eg. after electrical injury) In such cases, options include a tensor fascia latae, anterolateral thigh, or rectus femoris muscle flap. Various permutations of rectus abdominis muscle flaps are very useful for coverage of large defects around the groin, proximal thigh, external genitalia, and perineum.

Perineum

Perineal contractures are relatively rare, but can be very unpleasant and difficult to treat if severe.

Simple linear bands bridging across between the proximal thighs, vulva, penis or anus, can be released with Z plasties or Y–V plasties, as local flaps in this area tend to be relatively well vascularized.

For more severe contractures, a defunctioning colostomy should be considered as part of the management. Extensive grafting (split skin) is often required, and tie-over dressings are usually necessary because of the difficult contour. It is often helpful to mesh the grafts to optimize take.

Gracilis muscle is simple to elevate and very useful for coverage of defects around the genitalia and perianal area.

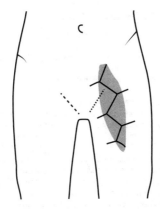

Fig. 30.13 For broadband contractures, local flaps from the groin, hypogastric area or thigh may be useful, if the area scarred is not very extensive. However, most often for broadband contractures in the groin, scarring is extensive and an extensive release and split skin graft is required (as the defect is commonly large, full thickness grafts are not often indicated in this site). Split skin grafts commonly do fairly well. Dermal substitutes may be useful in this area.

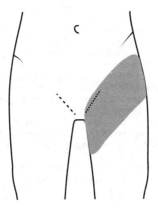

Fig. 30.14 Diffuse broadband flexion contracture at hip suitable for release and skin graft or dermal regeneration template.

Popliteal fossa and knee

The popliteal fossa is a common site for contracture after burns of the lower limb.

For linear band contractures a wide variety of options are available. Multiple Y–V plasties or Z plasties are the simplest options for relatively mild bands with some skin laxity. For thicker bands a local flap of propeller flap style may be used, but the donor site often cannot be sutured directly, so a skin graft is commonly required for the donor site.

For broadband contractures, skin grafts or flaps are required; it is often useful to use either a trapezoid flap release or two incisional releases proximal and distal to the joint to prevent making a deep incisional release into the popliteal fossa.

If a deep incisional release into the popliteal fossa is required, the popliteal vessels may be exposed. In this event a fasciocutaneous or perforator based propeller flap may be turned to cover the fossa, as long as reasonably scar-free skin is present either in the proximal calf (the medial or lateral distal thigh may also be used for a distally based flap). These flaps are also very useful for more moderate contractures as they put a 'fire-break' of normal skin in to break up the contracture and place the skin graft on the donor site on the side of the limb where contraction of the graft is not such an issue (Fig. 30.15).

In the rare event of the popliteal vessels being exposed and no skin flap being available, it is straightforward to turn up one of the gastrocnemius muscles to cover the popliteal fossa and create a safe graftable defect. If this has to be done as a turnover with the tendon facing superficially, the tendon should be excised to produce an optimum bed for a graft.

In the most severe contractures, requiring flaps, large skin grafts may be required to close all the defects. The bed for these grafts is often of irregular contour and a mesh graft is the best option to ensure good graft take.

Full correction of knee flexion contractures is important as subtotal corrections, leaving the knee flexed, usually result in recurrent contracture. Try hard to get full extension at the time of surgery, but if complete knee extension is not possible postoperatively then as soon as the graft or flap has healed it is important to consider further serial casting to gain full extension or gradual correction using the Ilizarov principle using an external fixator.

As with most joints contracture, postoperative splinting and physiotherapy are essential parts of the treatment.

The anterior knee is not often a site of a functional contracture per se, but may commonly be a site of an unstable scar with underlying superficial infection of patella. Debridement and flap repair is sometimes necessary if this fail to heal. The typical option for repair of this is a medial gastrocnemius muscle flap covered by a split skin graft. In addition, many useful skin flaps also exist for coverage of the anterior knee.

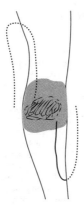

Fig. 30.15 Polpiteal fossa contracture may be released with proximally or distal based flaps raised predominantly sub facially. Avoid raising the proximally based flap from over the common peroneal nerve on the lateral aspect of knee. If a large perforator is in the base the flap can be islanded.

The foot and ankle

Dorsum

Dorsal foot contractures are very common. Hyperextension deformities of the metatarsophalangeal joints (MTPJs) of the foot result, and if the deformity is chronic, especially in adults, surgery to release the dorsal capsule of the MTPJ and lengthen the extensor hallucis longus may be necessary.

Minor contractures may be released with Y–Vs for linear bands. Often incisional release and skin grafting is required, because there is very little skin laxity on the dorsum of the foot.

When planning a release with skin grafting, it is best to place the transverse release incision proximally, about half way up the dorsum of the foot, so that when release occurs, the distal scarred skin of the dorsum still covers the MTPJ. This enables these joints to be released surgically and the extensor longus to be lengthened if required, while still leaving a graftable defect (rather than exposed joint/tendon which would need a flap).

Thick skin grafts or dermal substitutes are good options for the dorsum of the foot.

Occasionally, if extensive bone and joint work is required, a thin free flap may be necessary, but it can be challenging to obtain flap tissue that is thin enough to readily fit in a shoe (Fig. 30.16).

For major longstanding deformities, it is important to gauge function of the foot and ankle. Not uncommonly there can be secondary fixed deformity and even growth disturbance of the bones. Commonly toes are hyperextended and the MTPJs may be dislocated. In such circumstances be aware that skin contracture release alone may not effect a full correction or a functional foot. Even if full correction is attainable, accommodative orthoses may be necessary to allow weight bearing. Consider X-rays of foot and ankle to gauge deformity. Further bony surgery and open joint relocations or fusions may be necessary. If the patient has not been weight bearing at all for more than two years, then consideration needs to be given to ablative surgery in order to best regain function. Discuss with orthopaedic surgeons/orthotists/prosthetists if possible.

After an extensive incisional release it is often best to excise the skin edges as these are commonly of poor vascularity on the foot

K wiring in plantar flexion is extremely important after release of significant dorsal contractures. Typically the wires are left until the grafts are stable (about 4–5 weeks).

Commonly a broadband contracture of the dorsum of the foot is associated with a linear contraction of the dorsum of the ankle. In this event, a skin graft release is combined with a proximal Y–V or Z plasty.

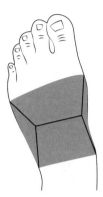

Fig. 30.16 Diagram showing incision for release of dorsal foot contracture placed at about mid-foot level so that the MTPJs are covered by intact skin when the release is carried distally. This allows grafting of the defect. Extensor brevis tendons can be excised if necessary. Often some skin has to be excised to prevent scar necrosis at the edges of the skin graft.

Sole and tendo achilles

Fortunately, contractures of the plantar surface of the foot are uncommon. They can readily be released with full thickness grafts in most cases, but grafts and marginal scars tend to produce troublesome hyperkeratosis that needs continuous treatment to alleviate discomfort.

Orthotists and podiatrists are invaluable specialists in looking after patients with post burn sole of foot problems, as surgery commonly does not satisfactorily resolve symptoms from scars on the sole.

Occasionally, equinus contractures can cause severe problems with mobility. Release with tendon lengthening is likely to require a free flap. An alternative is an ankle fusion or a 'pseudo fusion' with sacrifice of the tendo Achilles in patients with lower demands: this produces improved position of the foot at the expense of loss of powerful plantar flexion.

Conclusion

- Assess the contracture as well as possible. Remember it is a deficit of skin
- Release through the entire subcutaneous scar
- If the contracture is not releasing well, excise more scar
- If you are skin grafting, excise all subcutaneous scar to make a good bed
- Look after your patients well. They have already suffered much and they may need many more operations

Further reading

Hyakusoku H, Orgill DP, Teot L, et al. Colour atlas of burn reconstructive surgery. Heidelberg: Springer, 2010.
Shokrollahi K, Whitaker IS, Nahai F. Flaps: practical reconstructive surgery. Stuttgart: Thieme, 2017.

Outpatient management of minor burns

Introduction to outpatient management of minor burns

More than 90% of burns can be managed as outpatients by non-specialists, eg. emergency departments, minor injury units, and general practice. In practice, most burns are, at least, discussed with a burn service which then elects for outpatient management by either the burn service itself or non-specialists services for the lowest risk injuries. Outpatient management in supportive home environments aims to reduce unnecessary admissions and improve cost effectiveness without compromising quality of care. Although the majority of burns patients can be managed as outpatients, research has largely focused on burns requiring inpatient resuscitation, reducing high level evidence on which to base recommendations. This chapter summarizes widely accepted practice and existing evidence for consideration and does not constitute dogmatic recommendations.

Definition of minor burns

Various definitions of minor burns have been advanced. The following features are generally accepted:
- Limited extent (<3–5% total body surface area (TBSA)) and not requiring resuscitation
  - Superficial and superficial-partial thickness burns
  - ≤1% TBSA full-thickness burns in children or adults without cosmetic or functional risk to eyes, face, hands, feet, or perineum

Assessment and selection of patients for outpatient management

There are no internationally accepted criteria for selecting patients for outpatient management. The criteria in Table 31.1, expanded below, serve as a guide to features from the history and examination that should be considered.

- Age: patients at the extremes of age have intrinsically poorer outcomes. However, outpatient management may be suitable for all ages in select cases
- Comorbidities: cardiovascular, respiratory, neuropsychiatric, metabolic/renal, and endocrine systems may complicate outpatient management
- Social circumstances: including employment, distance and access to clinics should be ascertained. For example:
  - A child or adult who may have sustained their burn injury in questionable circumstances (eg. non-accidental injury) may be best managed initially as an inpatient with Social Services input
  - Patients managed as outpatients may be required to attend regular follow up appointments. It is important that selected patients have access to transport
  - An elderly patient living alone may not have family/friends to assist with care and may be best managed in hospital
- Severity/extent of injury: minor burns (see definition above) can usually be managed successfully as outpatients. However, some patients with comorbid renal failure, alcohol dependence, and patients in arid climates may require admission for intravenous fluid resuscitation even for minor burns
- Burn depth: while superficial burns usually heal within 3 weeks, full-thickness burns usually require admission for skin grafting. However, operative treatment for small burns can be performed on an outpatient or day case basis in a burns service. Where superficial partial thickness

Table 31.1 Factors to be considered when selecting patients for outpatient burn management

Patient factors	Age
	Comorbidities
	Social circumstances
Burn factors	Severity/extent of injury
	Depth
	Distribution
	Aetiology

Data sourced from Hartford CE, Kealey GP. Care of outpatient burns. In Herndon DN (ed.) Total burn care, 3rd edn. Edinburgh, UK: W.B. Saunders, pp. 67–80, Copyright © 2007, and Warner PM et al. Outpatient burn management. Surgical Clinics of North America 94(4):879–92, Copyright © 2014 Elsevier Inc. All rights reserved.

burns are managed as outpatients, these wounds should be regularly examined to identify conversion to deeper injuries and/or complications such as infections to allow early treatment

- Distribution: burn wounds on functionally and aesthetically sensitive areas such as the face, eyes, hands, and perineum may be need to initially be managed as inpatients because of potential difficulties relating to facial swelling, visual impairment, or difficulties in dressings
- Some burns in these anatomical regions, such as full thickness injuries traversing joint surfaces in the hands hands, may require early surgery to reduce the risk of debilitating contractures.
- Burn aetiology
  - Electrical burns: patients exposed to low voltage (<1 kV, although most household injuries are 120–220 V) can be considered for outpatient management if an electrocardiogram is normal or becomes normal during observation and if the wounds are small.
  - Chemical burns: it may be possible to manage some chemical burns as outpatients depending on location, extent, and depth. Rarely, large hydrofluoric acid burns necessitate inpatient treatment for monitoring of serum calcium levels and pain relief (see Chapter 19 Chemical burns). Poisons information services such as Toxbase (http://www.toxbase.org/) should be consulted
  - Flame burns: These are often deeper and can be associated with an inhalation injury. If the latter is suspected a full respiratory assessment should be performed and if present the patient should be managed as an inpatient in conjunction with Intensive Care Physicians.

First aid and initial management

- Cooling: cooling the burn wound for up to 20 minutes is an effective measure to dissipate heat and arrest tissue damage, stabilize mast cells and thus reduce oedema, and also has an analgesic effect. Cooling is most effective if commenced within 20–30 minutes of the injury. Cool tap water or soaks (8–25°C) may be used.
- Pain management: initial assessment and dressing of burns may require opioid analgesics. Adjuvants such as paracetamol and non-steroidal anti-inflammatory (NSAIDs) agents may also be used. Once a burn has been dressed, pain is usually manageable with oral analgesics such as NSAIDs or weak opioids. Patients usually require supplementary analgesia during dressing changes and physical therapy sessions. Patients with narcotic abuse or chronic pain issues may require specialist input. Anxiolytics such as benzodiazepines may also be required in certain cases
- Tetanus vaccination: tetanus vaccination status should be ascertained and boosters administered if required (see Chapter 39)

Local wound treatment

- Management of blisters: there is general agreement that these should be debrided to allow full assessment of depth and size. Very small, non-tense blisters may be left intact. Aspiration is not recommended as it may introduce infection without the benefit of the ability to fully assess the wound when fully deroofed.
- Cleansing and debridement: wounds may be cleansed with water, and/or mild non-irritant soaps. Debridement of wounds reduces the risk of infection and allows more accurate assessment of burn depth.
- Topical agents: there are a variety of topical agents used to dress burns. Examples include silver sulfadiazine and chlorhexidine. The latest Cochrane reviews have shown the evidence for these treatments to be generally weak, precluding evidence-based recommendations. Silver sulfadiazine has especially been consistently shown to be associated with poorer outcomes. The general principle should be to avoid use of these in clean, uncontaminated burns
- Wound dressings: a wide range of dressings is available including:
  • Simple dressings (fine mesh gauze, hydrocolloid, and silicone based)
  • Biosynthetic dressings (biobrane, biobrane-like dressings, and polyhexanide containing bio-cellulose). There is accepted evidence that Biobrane, when used in children with confluent superficial dermal burns within 48 hours of the injury, reduces the pain of subsequent dressing changes thereby enabling outpatient management in this patient group.
  • The 2013 Cochrane review, by Wasiak et al.,[1] assessing a range of dressings found that all 30 eligible studies were at risk of bias, precluding firm recommendations. In most small superficial burns simple non-adherent dressings combined with an absorbent layer will allow the wounds to heal spontaneously if changed every 2–4 days depending on the amount of exudate. Biologic and biosynthetic dressings may have some role in special areas such as the hand or in large burns to allow early movement, reduce exudate and pain, but are generally very rarely used in the outpatient setting.
- Management of itch: pruritus may affect >90% of burn sufferers in the first month. Suggested treatments are
  • First line: emollients should be used liberally to avoid dry skin, which may exacerbate pruritus
  • Second line: regular H1 receptor antagonists such as cetirizine are preferred over non-specific antihistamines such as diphenhydramine
  • Third line: neuropathic pain blockers such as gabapentin and pregabalin may be useful
  • Others: doxepin, massage therapy, and transcutaneous electrical nerve stimulation

Patient education

Successful outpatient management depends on motivated, informed patients. Patients should particularly be educated on:
- Pain management: patients should be advised to take additional analgesia during dressing changes and therapy sessions
- Features of infection: including fever, pain, and spreading redness/erythema. Parents of children should also be counseled to report any features of toxic shock syndrome including change in affect, dry nappies, rashes, abdominal pain, anorexia and any parental concern.
- Maintaining mobility: regular physical exercise of affected area, especially hands and feet, reduces the risk of stiffness or contractures if the burns are deep
- Elevation to reduce oedema: limbs, especially, should be raised to a level above the heart

Complications and when to admit

Patients initially managed as outpatients may require admission due to a number of possible complications including:
- Infection: there is no evidence supporting prophylactic antibiotics in burns since only 5% of patients managed as outpatients suffer infection. However, local or systemic infections should be treated aggressively according to local antibiotic policies. Microbiological culture of burn exudate may guide antibiotic selection. Swabbing of any burn before treatment for infection is essential. Any suspected cases of toxic shock syndrome should be managed expediently in collaboration with the receiving accident and emergency department, paediatricians, microbiologists, intensivists and the burns service.
- Delayed wound healing: this increases the risk of scarring and poor function/cosmesis. Some wounds may have progressed in depth and may require operative interventions such as skin grafting
- Social: patients failing to cope may require respite or inpatient care especially if other factors such as pain or difficult dressings are also of concern
- Uncontrolled or intractable pain
- Dressings: some body parts such as the perineum may be difficult to apply dressings or patients may have significant exudate requiring more frequent dressing changes

Follow-up

Follow-up arrangements vary depending on physician, institution, and patient preferences. However, intervals should be selected to ensure that adverse events, including conversion to deeper injuries, are promptly identified and rectified. Shorter intervals are preferred initially (commonly 2–3 days after the initial dressing then 3–7-day intervals), becoming longer if healing is satisfactory. Multidisciplinary clinics involving physiotherapists, occupational therapists and psychologists should be established to reduce patient inconvenience. Telemedicine may be appropriate for some patients. Outreach clinics may also reduce patient transportation costs and are an important way of following patients up.

Further reading

ISBI. Care of out patient burns. 2014. Available from http://www.worldburn.org/documents/burncare.pdf (accessed 2 July 2014).
Warner PM, Coffee TL, Yowler CJ. Outpatient burn management. Surgical Clinics of North America 2014;94:879–92.

Reference

Wasiak J, Cleland H, Campbell F, Spinks A. Dressings for superficial and partial thickness burns. Cochrane Database Syst Rev. 2013;28(3):CD002106.

Remote assessment of burns

Introduction to remote assessment of burns

Approximately 130,000 people with burn injuries visit Emergency Departments in the UK each year.[1] Of these approximately 12,000 are admitted to hospital. Around 6,000 children aged 0–15 years are admitted to hospital with burns (which equates to approximately 16 babies and children each day). Of these an average of 250 suffer a major burn (>10% total body surface area (TBSA) requiring fluid resuscitation.[2] The majority of cases referred to specialized burns services are not severe. However, even so, such injuries require specialized care to achieve good outcomes, reduce long-term scarring, and prevent other ongoing problems.

Organization of burn care in England and Wales

In England and Wales burn care is organized using a tiered model of care[2] where the most severely injured are cared for in 'Burns Centres' and those requiring less intensive clinical support being cared for in either a 'Burns Unit' or a 'Burns Facility'. This endeavours to provide a balance between easy access and care provided closer to home for the majority of patients with a smaller number of highly specialized centres for the smaller proportion of patients with more severe injuries.

There are four Adult Burns centres in England and Wales for Adults (Queen Elizabeth Hospital in Birmingham, Morriston Hospital in Swansea, Broomsfield Hospital in Chelmsford and Chelsea and Westminster Hospital in London) and four Childrens Burns centre (Birmingham Childrens Hospital, Queens Medical Centre in Nottingham, Frenchay Hospital in Bristol and Broomsfield Hospital in Chelmsford). This inevitably means a small subsection of patients with severe injuries potentially may need to travel long distances for management of their injuries.

Telemedicine

The World Health Organization (WHO) defines telemedicine (from the Greek prefix 'tele' meaning 'at a distance' and the Latin 'meden' meaning 'healing') as 'the delivery of health care services, where distance is a critical factor, by all health care professionals using information and communication technologies for the exchange of information for the diagnosis, treatment and prevention of disease and injuries, research and evaluation, and for the continuing education of health care providers in the interests of advancing the health of individuals and their communities.'[2]

Telemedicine is not a new branch of medicine or an activity aiming to replace health care workers and face-to-face consultations. Historically, it has been performed in a variety of ways, eg. postal services, telegraph, telephone, radio transmission, and initial video recording.

There are two main areas where it can be utilized effectively. Firstly, where there is no alternative, eg. in emergency situations in remote locations where medical care would be difficult or impossible to reach the patient in time. Secondly, where it improves the access to health service avoiding or reducing travel for patients or clinicians.

Modes of telemedicine

There are a number of different modes of telemedicine.[3]
- Store and forward or pre-recorded telemedicine (asynchronous). Information is acquired and stored in some format prior to being sent by appropriate means for expert consultation
- Realtime or video conference. There is no delay between the information being collected, transmitted, and displayed, and interactive communication between clinicians is possible
- Hybrid telemedicine. This involves is a combination of real-time and store and forward telemedicine techniques
- Mobile or cellular telemedicine. Portable devices with inbuilt camera (smartphones, laptops, tablets) capture digital images and computing and networking features allow digital interaction
- Integration model. Integration of electronic devices and software allows capturing, transferring, storage, measurement and delivery of follow-up

Medicolegal issues associated with telemedicine[4]

There have been many medicolegal and ethical concerns raised in regards to telemedicine including:
- The licensure
- Responsibilities and potential liabilities of the health professional
- Continuity of care
- Duty to maintain the confidentiality of patient records
- Informed consent
- Data security
- Jurisdictional problems associated with cross-border consultations
- Reimbursement of care provided by using a telemedicine service

Telemedicine in burns assessment and management

The severity of burn injuries is determined by the percentage of the TBSA injured and the depth of the burn. The injured body surface and depth of the burn wound are assessed mainly by visual inspection.

Over the past 40 years survival from burns injuries[5] has improved dramatically. Incidence has also decreased by more than half. However as incidence has decreased so has most physicians familiarity with burns assessment and treatment. Accuracy of burns assessment has been shown to be vastly increased when seen by a specialist and simple SAF telemedicine has been shown to be an effective method of assessment.[3,6] Recent advances in smart device technology have increased the potential to make this technology more accessible and cheaper but the informatics governance implications have lagged behind the technology.

Cost-effectiveness

There has been little evidence clearly demonstrating the cost-effectiveness of telemedicine in the assessment of burns injuries especially in developed countries. However, various projects have shown its clear advantage in both assessment and subsequent management, prevention of inappropriate or unnecessary referrals, and costly transfers to burns units.[3,5,7,8]

Conclusion[8]

Telemedicine has proved already to be a useful tool in Burns triage and is just beginning to be used more widely in trauma care, including plastic surgery, burns, neurosurgery, and orthopaedics. With work patterns changing and increasing super specialization within medicine, telemedicine may prove critical in helping to permit continued access to essential expertise.

Further reading

Claquinto-Cilliers MGC. Telemedicine, mobile phones and burn wound assessment: a valid resource for South Africa? Wound Healing Southern Africa 2013;6:56–9.

Saffle J, Edelman L, Theurer L, Morris S, Cochran AJ. Telemedicine evaluation of acute burns is accurate and cost-effective. Trauma, Injury, Infection and Critical care 2009;67:358–65.

Shokrollahi K, Sayed M, Dickson W, Potokar T. Mobile phones for the assessment of burns: we have the technology. Emergency Medicine Journal 2007;24:753–5.

Wallace DL, Jones SM, Milroy C, Pickford MA. Telemedicine for acute plastic surgical trauma and burns. Plastic and Reconstructive Aesthetic Surgery 2008;61:31–6.

Martin N, Lundy J, Rickard R. Lack of precision of burn surface area calculation by UK Armed Forces medical personnel. J Burns 2013.

Virendra Deo Sinha, Rahul Hath Tiwari, Rashim Kataria. Telemedicine in neurosurgical emergency: Indian perspective. Asain J Neurosurg. 2012;7(2):75–7.

Egol KA, Helfet DL, Koval KJ. Efficacy of telemedicine in the initial management of orthopaedic trauma. Am J Orthop (Belle Mead NJ) 2003;32(7):356–60.

References

1. NHS, Hospital Episode Statistics 2011 to 2012.
2. National Burn Care Review Committee Report, Standards and Strategy for Burn Care: A review of burn care in the British Isles, British Burn Association, February 2001.
3. Claquinto-Cilliers MGC. Telemedicine, mobile phones and burn wound assessment: A valid resource for South Africa? Claquinto-Cilliers MGC Wound Healing Southern Africa 2013;6(2):56–9.
4. Tsuchihashi Y, Okada Y, Ogushi Y, Mazaki T, Tsutsumi Y, Sawai T. The current status of medicolegal issues surrounding telepathology and telecytology in Japan. J Telemed Telecare 2000;6(suppl 1):143–5.
5. Saffle J, Edelman L, Theurer L, Morris S. Telemedicine evaluation of acute burns is accurate and cost-effective. Cochran A J Trauma, Injury, Infection and Critical care. 2009;67(2):358–65.
6. Shokrollahi K, Sayed M, Dickson W, Potoker T. Mobile phones for the assessment of Burns: we have the technology. Emerg. Med J 2007;24:753–5.
7. Wallace DL, Jones SM, Milroy C, Pickford MA. Telemedicine for acute plastic surgical trauma and burns. Plast Reconstr Aesthet Surg. 2008;61(1):31–6.
8. Wallace D, Hussain A, Khan N, Wilson Y. A systematic review of the evidence for telemedicine in burn care: with a UK perspective. Burns 2012;38:465–80.

Cost of burn care

Introduction to cost of burn care

The burden of burn injury, however trivial it may seem, is devastating physically, psychologically, and also financially. Health economists find it difficult to quantify the costs of acute care and almost impossible to define the cost of the needed adjustment after recovery. Burns patients often require long-term therapy and outpatient hospital care, and, frequently, re-admission for reconstructive surgery.

Calculating the cost of burn care is important for reimbursement, resource allocation and achieving efficiency by prudent cost analysis. Realistic cost estimates of burn care require robust data collection and a reliable informatics infrastructure.

Acute care cost

Staffing, operating theatre, intensive care, wound dressings, and the emerging new expensive technologies including skin substitutes are the most expensive categories in burns care. The operating theatre costs between £18 and £50 per minute depending on case complexity.[1] The first 2 days after admission to the burns or the critical care unit cost the most (equivalent of £6,650 day 1, £4,100 day 2, and £3,000 day 3). This is a reflection of the cost incurred till the patient is resuscitated and stabilized.[2] Skin substitutes including cultured cells technologies and cadaveric skin costs on average £5.50/cm² area covered. Mathew Klein[3] estimated the overall average cost of a paediatric burns to be £5,500, but costs will vary depending on country and healthcare systems. The severity of the burn—extent and depth— were the only two factors associated with a greater costs. One per cent of TBSA grafted increased the cost by £1,600 in one study.[3] On the other hand, it is estimated that the cost of acute care for a massive burn in the UK ranges from £500,000 to £1,000,000, excluding the rehabilitation costs, costs of social re-integration, and opportunity costs to society.[4]

Rehabilitation cost

The latest iteration of the UK burn care standards require off-site rehabilitation outside the acute care facility, yet the availability of rehabilitation facilities have yet to catch up with the standards, and commissioning of these facilities is not streamlined. The cost of rehabilitation includes loss of productive manpower, earnings, opportunities, and also the cost of social care and benefits. The impact of burns on the patient's family and carer has to be also taken into account. The long-term impact of the burn on the quality of life has been widely reported. However, there is very little related to the cost impact, and those funding rehabilitation are focusing increasingly on outcome measures. The World Health Organization's Global Disease Burden project has included fire as one of 107 major diseases. The disability-adjusted life years (DALYs) was used as a single measure for combined morbidity and mortality of a certain disease. The estimated DALYs per 100,000 population in Japan in 2004 for flame burns were 16 years, 28 for the USA, 209 in the Russian Federation, 461 in India, and 14 in the UK. However, the source data need more refining to produce a standardized comparative risk assessment tool.[5]

Cost containment

A cost containment programme is achieved by robust data collection, updated treatment protocols, outcomes and quality assurance measures, and lastly optimizing resources. In practice early surgical excision and modulation of the hypermetabolic response were shown to improve outcomes and reduce hospital stay. This is an excellent example of evidence-based cost containment. Lack of evidence-based medicine in burn care is a major factor that contributes to the increasing cost of burn care as new products and technologies are produced. Research can provide the tools that enable us to achieve better outcomes and cost efficiency.[6]

Prevention programmes in developed and developing countries should be regarded as the most cost containment programme in burn care.

Further reading

Barret JP. Cost-containment and outcome measures. In Herndon DN. Total burn care, 4th edn. London: WB Saunders 2012;707–14.

Klein MB, Hollingworth W, Rivara FP, et al. Hospital costs associated with pediatric burn injury. Journal of Burn Care Research 2008;29:632–7.

References

1. Macario A. What does one minute of operating room time cost? Journal of Clinical Anesthesia 2010;22:233–6.
2. Dasta JF, McLaughlin TP, Mody SH, Piech CT. Daily cost of an intensive care unit day: the contribution of mechanical ventilation. Critical Care Medicine 2005;33:1266–71.
3. Klein MB, Hollingworth W, Rivara FP, et al. Hospital costs associated with pediatric burn injury. Journal of Burn Care & Research. 2008;29:632–7.
4. Hemington-Gorse SJ, Potokar TS, Drew PJ, Dickson WA. Burn care costing: the Welsh experience. Burns 2009;35:378–82.
5. WHO. Health statistics and information systems. Estimates for 2000–2012. Disease burden. http://www.who.int/healthinfo/global_burden_disease/estimates/en/index2.html (accessed 27 September 2015).
6. Pruitt BA Jr, Wolf SE. An historical perspective on advances in burn care over the past 100 years. Clinics in Plastic Surgery 2009;36:527–45.

Paediatric burns

Introduction to paediatric burns

According to the World Health Organization, there are about 180,000 deaths from burns per year worldwide,[1] and 96,000 of these occur in children. Children are particularly vulnerable to burns, and infants are at a greatest risk. House fires are among the leading causes of burn-related deaths in children. Scalds are common in children less than 3 years old.

The many physiological differences between children and adults, in addition to anatomical differences, must be considered in the care of pediatric burn patients.

Initial evaluation

- Immediately remove child from the source of burn
- Remove clothing and jewellery, as these can prolong the burning process
- Avoid pouring cool water onto the burn in cases of large burns
- Cover child with a blanket or sheet to keep warm
- Irrigate chemical burns with a copious amount of water for at least 30 minutes
- Identify and treat any potential life-threatening traumatic injuries

Airway

- The airway should be assessed first
- Administer 100% oxygen and obtain arterial blood gas and carboxyhaemoglobin level if inhalation injury is suspected
- Stridor and hoarseness indicate an imminent airway crisis due to inhalation injury or oedema, and immediate intubation should be considered

Chest burn

- Circumferential full-thickness chest burn can impede chest expansion
- If ventilation is compromised, escharotomy of the chest should be performed

- A urinary drainage catheter is essential for burns >20%
- Nasogastric tube placed in major burns
- Burn size and depth determined promptly

Resuscitation

IV access
- Should be established immediately
- Peripheral IV access preferred
- May go through burned skin if needed
- Consider suturing IV lines
- Central venous line when peripheral IV not attainable

Intraosseous line
- When vascular access not available
- Fluid administration via intraosseous line can be performed in all children
- Proximal tibia most common site

Fluid losses
- Proportionally greater in children due to their small body weight-to-body surface area ratio
- Normal blood volume in children approximately 80 mL/kg body weight and 85–90 mL/kg in neonates

Burn size
- 'Rule of nines' is useful in adults but does not accurately reflect the burned body surface area of children under 15 years of age
- Lund–Browder chart is more accurate way of determining burn size in children

Resuscitation formulas
- Common resuscitation formulas are mostly weight-based and have been developed using adult patients
- Use of weight-based resuscitation formulas in children results in under- or over-resuscitation
- Pediatric burn patients should be resuscitated using formulas based on body surface area
- One formula uses 5,000 mL/m^2 total body surface area (TBSA) burned for resuscitation fluid plus 2,000 mL/m^2 TBSA for maintenance fluid given over the first 24 hours after burn
- Half the volume is administered during the initial 8 hours, and the second half is given over the next 16 hours
- Over the subsequent 24 hours, 3,750 mL/m^2 TBSA burned for resuscitation fluid plus 1,500 mL/m^2 TBSA for maintenance fluid should be used.

Estimation of the amount of fluid required
- Amount of resuscitation fluid should be titrated according to the patient's response
- Lactated Ringer's solution is the most commonly used resuscitation fluid for the first 24 hours after burn
- Fluid boluses, if indicated, should be administered in amounts appropriate for the size of the child (20 mL/kg)
- Children under 1 year of age should also receive a separate maintenance fluid containing dextrose to prevent hypoglycaemia

Assessment of resuscitation

- Children have remarkable cardiopulmonary reserve
- They often do not show clinical signs of hypovolaemia until > 25% of the circulating volume has been lost and complete cardiovascular decompensation is imminent
- Hypotension and low urine output are late manifestations of shock in the pediatric patient
- Distal extremity colour, capillary refill, pulse pressure, and mental status reflect volume status

Capillary refill
- Indicator of volume status
- Decreased capillary refill suggests imminent cardiovascular collapse

Lactic acid and base deficit
- Measurement of lactic acid or arterial pH with base deficit is important in pediatric burn population, and reflect decreased tissue perfusion
- Correction of lactic acid or base deficit shows effective resuscitation

Urine output
- Assessed hourly
- Resuscitation fluid should be adjusted to achieve a urine output of 1 mL/kg/h in children and 2 mL/kg/h in infants

Over-resuscitation
- Must be avoided
- Can lead to pulmonary oedema, abdominal compartment syndrome, extremity compartment syndrome, and cerebral oedema

Evaluation and management of airways

- Airway evaluation and management given priority in pediatric patients
- Children are more prone to airway obstruction

Early intubation

- Considered when severe inhalation injury is present, a patient has a large burn and is likely to develop airway oedema with a large amount of fluid resuscitation, or a long transfer is anticipated

Inhalation injury

- Any patient with flame burn, especially if confined in a closed space, should be evaluated for inhalation injury
- Signs of potential inhalation injury include facial burns, carbonaceous sputum, singed nasal hair, respiratory distress such as hoarseness, stridor, dyspnoea, wheezing, or altered mental status
- If inhalation injury is suspected, patient should be placed on 100% oxygen
- Arterial blood gas and carboxyhaemoglobin level should be obtained
- The initial carboxyhaemoglobin level should be calculated from the time the admission level is drawn back to the time of the burn injury using a nomogram.
- The definitive method of diagnosis is direct visualization of the airway with bronchoscopy

Treatment modalities for inhalation injury

- Airway maintenance, clearance, and pharmacological management
- Mainly supportive and includes humidified air, pulmonary toilet, and ventilator support if necessary
- Nebulized heparin and N-acetylcysteine have shown to decrease reintubation rates and mortality

Hypermetabolism

- Children with large burns demonstrate a profound hypermetabolism
- Prolonged hypermetabolism can lead to marked loss of lean body mass and increased morbidity and mortality
- Marked upregulation of catabolic agents leads to increased energy expenditure; loss of lean body mass and body weight; delayed wound healing; and immune depression
- Pharmacological agents have been used to attenuate hypercatabolism in burn injury
- Attenuation of lean body mass loss can be achieved in paediatric burn patients by administration of anabolic hormones such as recombinant human growth hormone and insulin; anabolic steroids such as synthetic testosterone analogue oxandrolone; and adrenergic antagonists such as propranolol

Nutrition

- Nutrition is an important part of treatment in pediatric burns
- Patients with >30% TBSA burns are placed on enteral tube feeding to supplement oral nutrition
- Patients with smaller burns are placed on a high-protein, high-calorie diet

Early enteral nutrition

- Provides nutritional support in hypermetabolic children with severe burns
- Can lessen the hypermetabolic response
- Improves intestinal blood flow and motility, and preserves gut mucosal integrity
- Enteral nutrition can be initiated within a few hours of admission

Formulas

- Several formulas are available to estimate caloric requirements in burned children
- Caloric support is given in amounts calculated based on body surface area in children as caloric demands are related to burn size
- A series of formulas based on body surface area are available to meet the differing requirements of various age groups
- One formula uses 1,500 kcal/m^2 TBSA burned plus 1,500 kcal/m^2 TBSA
- Commercially available enteral formulas are hyperosmolar and should be diluted to 1/2–3/4 strength because of the high incidence of diarrhoea in burned children.

Thermoregulation

- Infants and toddlers are particularly susceptible to hypothermia
- Extensive heat loss occurs after major burn through convection and evaporation
- Energy demands and evaporative water losses can be reduced by maintaining ambient temperatures at 30–33°C and humidity at 80%

Management of burn wounds

Topical antimicrobials
- The most commonly used treatment in partial-thickness burns
- Use can be painful during dressing change

Long-term dressing
- For partial-thickness burns, dressings such as silver-impregnated dressings can be applied
- Application of silver-impregnated dressings leads to less pain and shorter hospitalizations than topical antimicrobial
- Most silver-impregnated dressings on partial-thickness burns can be left on for up to 7 days and reduce pain associated with dressing changes

Early surgical excision and grafting
- Reduces the incidence of wound infection and sepsis
- Leads to decreased length of hospital stay and reduced mortality

Pain management

- Children do not always express their pain in the same way as adults
- Children may display pain through anxiety, agitation, depression, withdrawal, and regression

Morphine sulfate
- One of the most commonly used analgesics in paediatric burn patients
- Given intravenously

Fentanyl oral
- Used effectively for dressing change and wound care (10 µg/kg)
- Outpatients treated with hydrocodone/paracetamol or other oral opioid derivatives
- Some require addition of longer-acting narcotics such as methadone or morphine sulfate controlled release
- Other analgesics include intranasal remifentanil and sufentanil
- Anxiolytics such as dexmedetomidine, midazolam, and diazepam can be used as adjuncts

Reference

1. WHO factsheet 365. 2018. http://www.who.int/mediacentre/factsheets/fs365/en. Accessed 2 October 2018).

Non-accidental injury (NAI) in children

Introduction to NAI in children

Children are inquisitive and as a result, accidents may occur. Unfortunately children are vulnerable to non-accidental burn injuries.

Prevalence

- Non-accidental burns represent between 1% and 16% of all burns in children presenting to hospital.
- Deliberately inflicted burns are seen in 10% of physically abused and 5% of sexually abused children.
- Mortality due to non-accidental burns is higher than in accidental burns (5.6–9.6% vs. 2.6–6%).

Assessment

History

Details of injury must be meticulously gathered:

- Time of injury, mode, and sequence of events plus any first aid procedures undertaken must be clarified
- Is the history plausible? Is the history consistent?
- History should be reviewed repeatedly to check for variation, which may indicate an attempt to conceal a NAI
- Does the distribution of the injury fit in with known patterns of injury?

Examination

- ABCDs should be assessed and treatment provided according to ATLS protocol.
- Accurate and systematic examination of the patient's body should be performed in a warm and comfortable environment
- Size, site, and depth of burns should be recorded
- Photographs aid recording along with recording on burn charts
- Other injuries and bruises should be noted
- A chaperone should be present to ensure patient comfort and provide protection for the examining health professional

The assessment of NAI is undertaken by the multidisciplinary team including general practitioners, paediatricians, plastic surgeons, and emergency physicians, as well as nursing staff (paediatric, emergency, and school nurses) health visitors, and social workers. The police may need to be involved also.

Parents' and children's characteristics

- Parents may appear angry, abusive, or depressed and withdrawn
- They present late and may not be keen to allow their child to be assessed or admitted for treatment
- They may discharge their children before treatment is completed
- Parents of accidentally burnt children are very keen for medical attention. They present early to emergency services and are clearly upset and feel guilty about the burn
- Abused children are often withdrawn, anxious, or rebellious
- Older children may avoid talking about their injuries

Patterns of NAI

In order to detect NAI, health professionals must consider the possibility and therefore be vigilant. There are certain patterns of injury that should increase suspicion:

- Symmetrical 'glove and stocking' scalds and buttock scalds with 'doughnut sparing' of the perineum are characteristic of forced immersion injuries. The doughnut sparing occurs due to the perineum coming into contact with the base of the bath and the hot water producing scalds to the other areas
- Non-accidental burns have uniform burn depth and well-delineated upper margins; accidental burns are varied in depth and have irregular upper margins
- Symmetrical scalds should be treated with great suspicion as a child would never enter a bath with both feet simultaneously
- Branding in the shape of the hot objects pressed against the skin leave tale tell marks. Common objects used include spoons and forks
- Cigarette burns produce a deep circular crater with or without a more superficial tail (caused as the cigarette moves against the skin after initial contact). They may be single or multiple
- Burns may be multiple and of varying age. This should further evoke suspicion

Differential diagnosis

It is important to keep an open mind. Occasionally a lesion may not be due to abuse. If there is no history of burn and the history is plausible and consistent then alternative diagnoses should be considered.

- Impetigo, epidermolysis bullosa, urticarial, contact dermatitis, and severe nappy rash may mimic a burn injury
- Freak accidents do occur. Burns secondary to seatbelt straps on a very hot day *do* occur. Likewise vinegar (acetic acid) is acidic (pH 1–2) and so prolonged contact could lead to a chemical burn
- If a child has a neurological deficit then the normal protective mechanisms will not prevent burn injuries. In these situations unusual accidental burns may occur

Health professionals must not overlook neglect. Children may present with burns as a result of neglect (negligent inability to protect a child from injury). Although the burn injury is not deliberately inflicted as in abuse, the incident should serve a warning of potentially devastating injury. It is therefore our duty as health professionals to report these incidents to appropriate authorities to minimize future risk.

Further reading

Andronicus M, Oates RK, Peat J, Spalding S, Martin H. Non-accidental burns in children. Burns 1998;24:552–8.

Greenbaum A, Donne J, Wilson D, Dunn KW. Intentional burn injury: an evidence based, clinical and forensic review. Burns 2004;30:628–42.

Maguire S, Moynihan S, Mann M, Potokar T, Kemp AM. A systematic review of the features that indicate intentional scalds in children. Burns 2008;34:1072–81.

Chapter 36

Burns itch

Introduction to burns itch

- Post-burn pruritus is one of the most common and distressing complications of burn injury
- Itching typically begins in the first 2 weeks after burn injury and may last for an extended period of time (several years)
- Post-burn pruritus may interfere with
  - Sleep
  - Activities of daily living
  - May complicate healing when scratching damages healing or thin epithelium and newly grafted skin
  - Can cause problems with concentration and lead to depression

Definition

Itch was initially described in 1660 by Samuel Hafenreffer, a German physician who defined itch as an 'unpleasant sensation that elicits the desire or reflex to scratch.' This definition remains the most used.

Types of pruritis

- Itch is arbitrarily divided into acute and chronic with the transition occurring at 6 months following onset of symptoms. The other categorization is based on location of the origin of the itch experience
  - Pruritogenic: localized to the skin and associated with dryness, inflammation or other cutaneous injury (the type most associated with burn injuries)
  - Neuropathic: due to dysfunction along the peripheral nerve pathway
  - Neurogenic: itch arising due to central nervous system dysfunction without evidence of peripheral pathology
  - Psychogenic: the experience of itch in the absence of any organic pathology

Causes which increase itch

Injury type

- All mechanisms of burn injury can lead to itch; however, scald injury is most common followed by flame or contact injuries

Location

- Legs are most commonly affected by itch followed by the arms and then the face

Surgical Intervention

- Grafted burns are at greater risk of developing itch than non-grafted burns. This may be a function of time to healing and burn depth.
- The presence of itch correlates positively with number of surgical procedures
- Wounds requiring more than 3 weeks to heal

Burn Surface area involved

- > 40% TBSA is associated with increased itching

Itch also correlates positively with PTSD symptoms and poor coping strategies

Environmental

- High ambient temperature (70%) and/or sweating (61%)
- Skin dryness (83%)
- Stress and fatigue (57%) increase itch
- Movement (52%) can increase itch
- Particular fabrics (48%)
- For some subjects, cold temperatures (30%), cold water (26%), and rest (22%) helped combat itch symptoms

Epidemiology

- 87–100% incidence following burn injury
- Onset at 1 month with peak symptoms at 6 months
- One study reported 87% incidence at 3 months, 70% at 12, and 67% at 24 months. In another study, at 4 years post injury, 79% of patients reported some problems with itch and in 29% this was persistent. At 12 years this figure reduced to 44% and 5%, respectively
- Gender distribution is female > male

Biology (neurotransmitters involved in itch)

- Histamine from mast cells and keratinocytes bind a variety of histamine receptors
  - H1 neuroreceptors are most associated with itch these are located on the unmyelinated C fibre peripheral nerves
  - H2 (peripheral nerves), H3 (central), and H4 (mast cells) may have a role
- Acetylcholine from skin cells and autonomic synapses and binds cutaneous muscarinic receptors
- Kinins including neurokinin A and bradykinin bind vanilloid receptors (VR-1) on the C fibres. Vanilloid receptors are likely to be antagonistic to itch mediators
- Substance P binds the neurokinin-1 receptor (NK-1) on C fibres
- Proteinases; tryptase and mast cell chymase bind proteinase activation receptor (PAR-1) on the C fibre
- Following burn injury there is an initial depletion of cutaneous mast cells, substance P positive nerve fibres, proteinases, and inflammatory mediators; at 2 weeks the levels are increased significantly over pre-injury levels

Biology

Itch neurological pathways

- Specific unmyelinated C fibres synapse in the dorsal horn signals travel orthodromically in the spino-thalamic tract to the thalamus then on to the somatosensory cortex (areas in the cingulate gyrus and prefrontal cortex connections are also activated explaining the emotional response)
- There is evidence for localized antidromic signally leading to a histamine releasing positive feedback loop

Assessment

Objective assessment of itch is difficult and uses experimental techniques like perceptual matching, MRI/PET, microneurography and accelerometers to measure itch while asleep. Itch is a subjective experience; however, many factors influence the intensity of itch at the point of observation. Commonly used and accepted techniques include:

- Visual analogue scale with a range 0–10 anchored between no itch and worst possible itch
- The 'Itch Man Scale' copyrighted by the Shriners Hospitals based on the Likert 5-point scale
- Itch Severity Scale developed by Yosipovitch based on the Modified McGill Pain Scale
- The itch component of the Abbreviated Burns Specific Health Scale

Therapy for itch

Adults and children can use the same interventions for the management of itch with adjusted dosing for weight and age and observing for unwanted side effects.

- Simple interventions which compliment the pharmacological interventions include
  - Moisturisers: simple (E45/Nivea), Aloe-Vera
  - Cooling, rest, the provision of appropriate environment (place, lighting, noise, temperature, décor, etc.), reassurance, distraction, imagery and relaxation techniques
  - Non-irritant garments
  - Silicone scar therapy
- First-line pharmacological therapy involves antihistamines
  - First generation: chlorpheniramine, diphenhydramine, hydroxyzine, cyproheptadine bind histamine, muscarinic, alpha-adrenergic, and serotonergic receptors and are sedative
  - Second generation: cetirazine, loratidine bind histamine receptors and inhibit leukotriene release
- Second-line pharmacological therapy involves
  - Gabapentin/pregabalin increasing dose until therapeutic effect achieved
  - Topical antihistamines; mepyramine, chlorpheniramine, hydroxyzine
  - Histamine H2 antagonist cimetidine
  - Capsaicin cream 0.025% (which works through neuropeptide depletion)
  - Topical dothiepin cream (5%) (Doxepin) some sedative effect but 50–800 better histamine binding that first-generation antihistamines.
- Adjuncts include
  - Massage
  - Psychological support
  - Transcutaneous nerve stimulation (TENS)
- Emerging or third-line techniques
  - Topical dapsone
  - Naltrexone (significant side effects)
  - Laser
  - Topical EMLA on small areas
  - Topical nano-crystalline silver

Nutritional requirements in the burn patients

Increased nutritional requirements after burns

Hypermetabolism can last for up to 36 months following burns, covering more than 30% of total body surface area (TBSA), raising calorie requirements up to 200% above baseline. Cachexia and lean muscle loss ensue, resulting in adverse outcomes. For example, losses in total body mass of 10%, 20%, 30%, and 40% can lead to immune dysfunction, decreased wound healing, severe infections, and death respectively. Therefore, alongside resuscitation, surgery and pharmacological measures (anabolic agents), nutritional supplementation is crucial in ameliorating hypermetabolism. It not only treats dietary deficiencies, but also supports healing and recovery.

Route and timing of feeding

Where feasible, nasogastric or nasojejunal enteral feeding is preferred for several reasons including reduced bacterial translocation and sepsis, increased splanchnic blood flow, and preservation of alimentary structure. For burns >20% TBSA, enteral tubes may be more appropriate than oral feeding as patients may have altered mentation, endotracheal ventilation, and require large volumes of feed to meet metabolic needs. Enteral nutrition should ideally commence within 12 hours post burn as this improves outcomes. Nasojejunal feeding reduces pneumonia rates, improves nutritional intake, and may be preferable. When safe, such as when post-burn ileus has resolved, the oral route may be used. Parenteral nutrition may be necessary where requirements cannot be met enterally. However, parenteral feeding is associated with overfeeding and a greater incidence of complications including catheter-related sepsis.

Energy requirements

Both over- and underfeeding can lead to poor outcomes. It is therefore crucial that supplementation closely matches requirements. Measurement of resting energy expenditure by indirect calorimetry remains the gold standard for assessing caloric requirements. However, since many centres do not possess calorimetric equipment, predictive equations are often used (Table 37.1). Only the recommended adapted Toronto equation correlates highly with indirect calorimetry but may be too complicated for routine clinical practice. Pragmatism may be required since controversy regarding the most accurate equation is ongoing.

Table 37.1 Daily calorific requirement estimation equations for adults and children

Equation	Patient Group	Requirement (kcal/day)
Galveston infant	0–1	2,100 kcal/m² + 1,000 kcal/m² burn
Galveston revised	1–11	1,800 kcal/m² + 1,300 kcal/m² burn
Galveston adolescent	12–16	1,500 kcal/m² + 1,500 kcal/m² burn
Toronto	Adults	−4,343 + (10.5 × %TBSA) + (0.23 × kcal) + (0.84 × Harris–Benedict) + (114 × temperature °C) – (4.5 × days after injury) *Where kcal = calorie intake in last 24 hours*
Schofield	Female 3–10 years	(16.97 × weight in kg) + (1,618 × height in cm) + 371.2
Schofield	Male 3–10 years	(19.6 × weight) + (1033 × height) + 414.9
Schofield	Female 10–18 years	(8,365 × weight) + (4.65 × height) + 200
Schofield	Male 10–18 years	(16.25 × weight) + (1372 × height) + 515.5
Curreri formula	16–59	25 kcal/kg of weight + (40) TBSA
Curreri formula	>60	20 kcal/kg of weight + (65) TBSA

Modified Harris–Benedict equation (for basal requirements without stress or activity allowance).

Male: BEE (kJ) = 278 + (57.5 × kg Wt) + (20.9 × cm Ht) – (28.3 v age).

Female: BEE (kJ) = 2741 + (40 × kg Wt) + (7.7 × cm Ht) – (19.6 × age).

Data sourced from Rousseau AF, et al. SPEN endorsed recommendations: nutritional therapy in major burns. Clinical Nutrition 32(4):497–502, Copyright © 2013.

Elsevier, and Rodriguez NA, et al. Nutrition in burns: Galveston contributions. Journal of Parenteral and Enteral Nutrition 35:704e14, Copyright © 2011 SAGE Publications.

Food types

Proteins

Patients with large burns, and without protein supplementation, usually have a negative protein balance due to proteolysis, which aims to provide substrates for gluconeogenesis. This contributes to cachexia and reduces immune function. Protein replacement is therefore a key goal of nutritional supplementation. Protein requirements of 1.2–2 g/kg/day and 2.5–4 g/kg/day are widely accepted as appropriate for burned adults and children respectively.

Glutamine, an immune-enhancing amino acid, is of particular interest but remains controversial. Although glutamine significantly reduces the incidence of Gram-negative bacteraemia and inpatient mortality, the duration of admission, wound infections, or the number of positive blood cultures are not affected. Further high-quality trials are required to further test the utility of glutamine in burns.

Carbohydrates

Glucose is the preferred fuel for metabolic pathways. Increased glucose requirements, secondary to hyperanabolism, increase the rate of carbohydrate hydrolysis potentially causing deficiency. Carbohydrate deficiency may lead to cachexia and proteolysis and therefore requires correction. Current guidelines advise delivering 55–60% of daily calorific requirements as carbohydrate without exceeding a 5 mg/kg/min limit for both adults and children.

Patients with large burns may be insulin resistant. Therefore, to maintain ICU-recommended blood glucose levels of 5–8 mmol/L, insulin may be required although the evidence for metformin and exenatide remains weak.

Lipids

Fat supplementation should be judicious. Post-burn lipolysis increased free fatty acids but 70% of this is re-esterified and may accumulate in the liver since hypermetabolism reduces fat utilization capacity. Evidence on which the recommendation to supply <35% of calorific requirements as fat is weak.

Vitamins and trace elements

Micronutrient deficiencies result in diminished skeletal, neuromuscular, and immune function. Micronutrient requirements are usually increased to levels where enteral nutrition alone becomes insufficient (Table 37.2).

Grade C evidence supports the recommendation to replace zinc, selenium, copper, and the vitamins B1, C, D, and E. However, early supplementation of high-dose vitamin C is not yet standard practice and the effect of vitamin D (400 IU/day) supplementation on osteoporosis incidence remains unclear.

Table 37.2 Reference daily intakes of micronutrients in burned patients

Age	Vitamin C, IU	Vitamin D, IU	Vitamin E, IU	Zinc, mg	Selenium, mg	Copper, mg
0–13	250–500	Unclear	Unclear	12.5–25	60–140	0.8–2.8
Over 13s	1000	Unclear	Unclear	25–40	300–500	4

IU, international units; mg, milligrams

Adapted with permission from Rodriguez NA, et al. Nutrition in burns: Galveston contributions. Journal of Parenteral and Enteral Nutrition 35: 704e14, Copyright © 2011 SAGE Publications. Source data: Dietary Reference Intakes for Calcium, Phosphorous, Magnesium, Vitamin D, and Fluoride (1977); Dietary Reference Intakes for Thiamin, Riboflavin, Niacin, Vitamin B6, Folate, Vitamin B12, Pantothenic Acid, Biotin, and Choline (1988); Dietary Reference Intakes for Vitamin C, Vitamin E, Selenium, and Carotenoids (2000); and Dietary Reference Intakes for Vitamin A, Vitamin K, Arsenic, Boron, Chromium, Copper, Iodine, Iron, Manganese, Molybdenum, Nickel, Silicon, Vanadium, and Zinc (2001). These reports may be accessed at http://www.nap.edu

Monitoring

Nutritional requirements vary throughout the post-injury period. Patients require vigilant multidisciplinary monitoring to avoid over- or underfeeding and identification of complications such as refeeding syndrome. Weight is regarded among the best indicators of nutritional status, and may be used alongside other indicators such as serum proteins and nitrogen balance. Feeding regimes which meet requirements can usually be prepared in liaison with pharmacy departments. Alternatively, there are several commercial formulas with varying concentrations of ingredients (see Rodriguez et al.[1]).

Further reading

Herndon DN, Tompkins RG. Support of the metabolic response to burn injury. Lancet 2004;36:1895–902.

Heyland, DK, Wischmeyer, P, Jeschke, MG, Wibbenmeyer, L, Turgeon, AF, Stelfox, HT, Day, AG, Garrel, D. A Randomized trial of ENtERal Glutamine to minimIZE thermal injury (The RE-ENERGIZE Trial): a clinical trial protocol. Scars, Burns & Healing 2017;3:2059513117745241.

Mosier MJ, Pham TN, Klein MB, et al. Early enteral nutrition in burns: compliance with guidelines and associated outcomes in a multicenter study. Journal of Burn Care & Research 2011;32:104–9.

Rousseau AF, Losser MR, Ichai C, Berger MM. ESPEN endorsed recommendations: nutritional therapy in major burns. Clinical Nutrition 2013;32:497–502.

Reference

1. Rodriguez NA, Jeschke MG, Williams FN, et al. Nutrition in burns: Galveston contributions. Journal of Parenteral and Enteral Nutrition 35:704e14.

Tetanus

Introduction to tetanus

Tetanus is the clinical manifestation of *Clostridium tetani* infection, a Gram-positive obligate anaerobic bacterium that exhibits spore-based transmission and is predominantly found in soil.[1,2] *Clostridium tetani* produces the exotoxin tetanospasmin, which blocks the inhibitory GABA pathway in the central nervous system; this results in unopposed reflex activity and ultimately the classical spasm pattern of trismus or 'lock jaw' that is associated with the infection.[1,2]

The childhood immunization programme introduced in the UK in 1961 has effectively eradicated tetanus in the UK; however, elderly people and those patients who have not completed a five-vaccine program of immunization remain at risk.[1,2]

Classifying tetanus-prone injuries

Tetanus-prone Injuries

- Injuries associated with sepsis and/or open fractures
- Puncture wounds or those containing foreign bodies
- A greater than 6-hour delay to theatre following trauma

Injuries with a high-risk of tetanus contamination

- Those occurring in immunocompromised patients
- Injuries associated with large volumes of devitalized tissue
- Heavy contamination with tetanus prone debris

Management

Prophylaxis

Tetanus toxoid IM injection (often a combination vaccine)
- Stimulates immunity by inducing antitoxin production
- Five injections are thought to confer lifelong immunity

Tetanus immunoglobulin IM injection
- Human immunoglobulin which neutralizes the exotoxin
- 500 international units (IU) is the standard dose in burns
- Bioavailability is achieved 2–3 days after injection and it has a 3–4 week half-life

Clinically apparent C. tetani infection
Tetanus is a clinical diagnosis. The cornerstones of treatment are antibiotics, surgical debridement and intensive care management. IM and intravenous immunoglobulin (IVIg) may be of use in neutralizing circulating exotoxin but they do not treat the existing spasm caused by tetanospasmin already bound to neurons[2] (Table 38.1).

Table 38.1 Tetanus prophylaxis regimen required in all wound types dependent upon previous immunization and associated risk of *Clostridium tetani* infection

Immunization history	Tetanus prophylaxis		
	Low risk or clean injury	Tetanus-prone injury	High-risk injury
5-year vaccination program complete	Nil required	Nil required	Immunoglobulin only*
Incomplete course or unsure of status	Toxoid booster**	Toxoid booster and immunoglobulin**	Toxoid booster and immunoglobulin**

*High-risk injuries require immunoglobulin treatment to neutralize the exotoxin regardless of the prior vaccination history.

**A full 5-vaccination course should be completed.

Data sourced from Department of Health. Tetanus. Chapter 30. In Immunisation against infectious disease: The Green Book, Public Health England, London, UK © Crown Copyright 2014, available from https://www.gov.uk/government/publications/tetanus-the-green-book-chapter-30. Reproduced under the Open Government Licence v3.0.

Tetanus is a preventable disease with a high associated mortality; with appropriate immunization, it could be eradicated entirely.

References

1. Cook TM, Protheroe RT, Handel JM. Tetanus: a review of the literature. British Journal Anaesthesia 2001;87:477–87.
2. Department of Health. Immunisation against infectious disease: the Green Book. Tetanus: Chapter 30. 2013. London: Public Health England.

Chapter 39

Desquamating skin disorders

Introduction to desquamating skin disorders

Also termed exfoliative and necrotizing diseases of the skin. Desquamation of the skin literally means shedding of the skin. In normal physiology desquamation of the keratinocytes occurs approximately every 14 days. Pathological desquamation involving skin and mucous membranes can cause significant morbidity and associated complications such as wound infection, sepsis, poor nutrition and pain, synonymous with a major burns patient.

Classification

- Scalded skin syndrome (SSS). Characterized by skin lesions limited to one mucosal surface
- Stevens Johnson syndrome (SJS). Two or more mucosal surface involvement in addition to systemic complications and involving less than 10% body surface area
- Toxic epidermal necrolysis (TEN). A more severe form of SJS affecting more than 30% body surface area. Between 10% and 30% the condition is frequently referred as SJS/TEN

Aetiology

This is an immunological reaction to a foreign antigen. It is usually iatrogenic, mainly involving the use of pharmacological agents. Antimicrobials, anticonvulsants, analgesics, NSAIDs, and corticosteroids have all been the culprit causing TEN. In addition to drugs viral illnesses have also been reported to cause such an immunological reaction to create SSS and SJS.

Clinical presentation

Signs and symptoms typically seen:
- A persistent pyrexia
- General malaise
- Cough
- The above may precede dermatological signs by up to 3 weeks

Following general symptoms patients present with generalized tender erythema. These progress to bullous eruptions. As the disease progresses vesicles and larger bullae emerge from erythematous areas. Erythema is followed by epidermolysis.

Nikolsky's sign is when the epidermis separates on gentle pressure of the skin surface: a sign showing the clinician desquamation of the skin. Sometimes there may be a lag period (1–3 weeks) from initial immunological insult (ie. administration of a drug) to skin eruption. The differential characteristics of SSS, SJS, and TEN are summarized in Table 39.1

Table 39.1 Clinical characteristics of desquamating skin disorders

	SSS	SJS	TEN
Preceding symptoms	None	Pyrexia, general malaise	Pyrexia, general malaise
Skin lesion distribution	Symmetrical, limbs	Variable; <10% TBSA	Diffuse; >30% TBSA
Character of skin lesions	Some target lesions	Vesicles; Nikolsky's positive	Epidermal detachment; no target lesions; large lesions; Nikolsky's positive
Biopsy features	Dermoepidermal separation with a mononuclear perivascular cell infiltrate with target lesions	A more intense dermal infiltrate than SSS	Minimal dermal inflammatory infiltrate and large areas of epidermal detachment
Mucosal involvement	One surface	Two or more	Two or more and severely affected
Recovery time	4 weeks	6 weeks	6 weeks
Mortality rate	0%	0–40%	25–80%

Pathology

A skin biopsy is crucial to identify the severity of the desquamation. The dermal infiltrates are made up of immunological cells including cytotoxic T-cells and T-helper cells. Dendritic lymphoid cells are also seen in addition to damaged dermal macrophages and necrotic keratinocytes. As seen in other inflammatory skin diseases there is a higher expression of HLA-DR on the keratinocytes. Immunofluorescence microscopy will reveal IgM antibodies and C3 along the dermoepidermal junction in SJS and TEN. The immune reaction of these disorders is said to be a type II cytotoxic reaction and type IV delayed hypersensitivity reaction.

Management outline

- TEN is a life threatening disease and thus a surgical emergency
- Admission to the burns unit
- Multidisciplinary team (MDT) approach

The role of the MDT

- Dermatology. Two punch biopsies to confirm TENS or SJS
- One biopsy in formalin, second in Michael's medium for immunofluorescence
- Treatments to skin made collaboratively with plastic surgery and dermatology
- Ophthalmology review early to assess for ocular therapy
- Anaesthesia and ICU teams to be involved at the time of referral or admission to assess for requirements of intubation

Initial assessment

- Observations 1–6 hourly including monitoring of airway. Include standard set of bloods including full blood count, urea and electrolytes, albumin, total protein
- Accurate medical and drug history and involve family and the patient's GP
- Precipitating symptoms such as fever, sore throat, conjunctival symptoms, general malaise
- Commence early analgesic regime
- Liaise with dermatology, may proceed with a skin biopsy
- Liaise with dietician and assess for nasogastric feeding
- Stress ulceration prophylaxis should be started and pulmonary support may require the input of the anaesthetic or intensivist team
- Corneal involvement can be common and should be managed with regular saline drops and early involvement of the ophthalmology team
- Assess severity using the SCORTEN scale
- As with major burns, these patients require aggressive fluid resuscitation, additional nutritional support, expert wound care, and a multidisciplinary approach involving physiotherapy, occupational therapy, dietician for nutritional support, and psychology
- Drugs suspicious of causing the reaction should be discontinued immediately

Further management

- Medical photography
- Daily multidisciplinary review
- Daily dressings to reduce risk of sepsis
- Clinical isolation
- Fluid and electrolyte balance
- Maintain peripheral IV access
- Anticoagulation prophylaxis

Wound management

- Swabs for microscopy, culture, and sensitivities
- Do not use prophylactic antibiotics as this may increase the risk of wound sepsis
- Dressings daily and review by the MDT

Surgical approach to management

- Debridement of necrotic epidermal tissue
- Coverage with a biological or synthetic dressings similar to those used in major burns. A particularly good indication for Biobrane
- Debridement of sloughed tissue will reduce the risk of sepsis from bacterial overgrowth
- Dressings will provide an analgesic effect over the tender exposed dermis
- In order to reduce bacterial overgrowth topical agents containing silver nitrate which may be present in dressings
- As these conditions are immunogenic, immunomodulating drugs such as corticosteroids, cyclosporine A, and intravenous immunoglobulin have been considered. Their use is controversial and these should not be commenced until discussion with the transferring or admitting burns unit

Prognosis

The SCORTEN system was introduced to predict mortality in patients with TENS and seven significant factors were identified:

- Age >40 years
- Evidence of cancer or haematological malignancy
- Tachycardia >120 beats/minute
- TBSA involvement at day 1 >10%
- Serum urea level >10 mmol/L
- Serum glucose level >14 mmol/L
- Serum bicarbonate level >20 mmol/L
  The probability of death is given by the formula:
  $P(death) = e^{logit}/1 + e^{logit}$
  where logit $= -4.448 + 1.237(SCORTEN)$
  Generally mortality rates are estimated (Table 39.2).

Table 39.2 Mortality rates

No of risk factors	Mortality rate
0–1	3.2%
2	12.1%
3	35.3%
4	58.3%
>5	>90%

Adapted from Bastuji-Garin S, et al. SCORTEN: a severity-of-illness score for toxic epidermal necrolysis. Journal of Investigative Dermatology 2000;155(2):149–53, Copyright © 2000.

The Society for Investigative Dermatology, Inc., with permission from Elsevier, http://www.jidonline.org/article/S0022-202X(15)40939-X/abstract.

Further reading

Bastuji-Garin S, Fouchard N, Bertocchi M, et al. SCORTEN: a severity-of-illness score for toxic epidermal necrolysis. Journal of Investigative Dermatology 2000;115:149–53.

Creamer D, Walsh SA, Dziewulski P, et al. U.K. guidelines for the management of Stevens–Johnson syndrome/toxic epidermal necrolysis in adults 2016. British Journal of Dermatology 2016;174:1194–227.

Guillaume JC, Roujeau JC, Revuz J, et al. The culprit drugs in 87 cases of toxic epidermal necrolysis (Lyell syndrome). Archives of Dermatology 1987;123:1166–70.

Yetiv J, Bianchini JR, Owens JA. Etiological factors in Stevens-Johnson syndrome. Southern Medical Journal 1980;73:599–602.

Military burns

History

The concept of a dedicated burn team and unit was established in 1940 by McIndoe at East Grinstead during the Battle of Britain.

Epidemiology

- 5% of all war casualties (troops and civilians) are burns,[1] 60% are accidental and 40% combat.[2] Combat burns are associated with greater Injury Severity Scores, full thickness burns, and inhalation injury[3]
- Mainly affects young males and exposed areas, eg. face and hands[3]
- The majority are ~5% TBSA,[4] Up to 25% are >20% total body surface area (TBSA)[5]

Causes

- Explosive weapons (main[5]). Ordnance devices produce fragments from the casing, Improvised explosive devices (IEDs) produce fragments from and within the casing and cause more burns[2]
- Incendiary weapons, eg. white phosphorous or napalm
- Chemical weapons. Can be lethal (eg. blistering) or incapacitating. Blistering agents cause burns, eg. mustard gas.
- Radiation or nuclear weapons
- Environment, eg. contact, scald, electrical, cold (frostbite)

General management

During triage >70% TBSA have expectant care, 20–70% TBSA +/– inhalation injury receive early evacuation, and <20% TBSA have delayed hospital care.[6]

- Levels of care include Level I Medical Support within the field, Level II Aid Station +/- surgical capability, Level III Field Hospital offering subspecialty care and Level IV Tertiary Burns Centre in home country. Most soldiers arrive back within 2–4 days[2]
- Resuscitation follows ATLS and EMSB/ABA guidelines including warming, IV crystalloid via the Parkland or modified Brooke formula,[7] IV antibiotics, and tetanus prophylaxis if associated contaminated battlefield wounds, and analgesia. Blisters are left intact until arrival in a clean environment and wounds are dressed[8] During evacuation chemical thromboprophylaxis is given and nasogastric tubes are placed for enteral feeding
- Early escharotomy is considered if deep circumferential burns prior to transport[8] but definitive surgery is performed early (<5 days post injury) in the burns centre

Burn infections

- Major organisms include Acinetobacter baumannii >Pseudomonas aeruginosa >Klebsiella pneumoniae >Staphylococcus aureus. For the first 15 days Acinetobacter and Staphylococcus predominate. After 15 days Pseudomonas and Klebsiella predominate[3]
- Topical antimicrobials dressings used include Mafenide acetate (Sulfamylon), Silver sulfadiazine (eg. Flamazine), silver nitrate solution, and silver-impregnated dressings (eg. Acticoat). Systemic antibiotics are given in infected wounds
- Infection associated mortality occurs at higher rates in combat burns. The main infections causing death include fungus (eg. *Aspergillus*), *Pseudomonas*, and *Klebsiella*[9]

Outcomes

- Gross functional outcomes are good and similar to civilians[3] but face and hand burns can lead to long-term physical and psychological morbidity[10]
- Mortality in military burns at the burn centre is ~4%, which is similar to civilians with same age range.[3] The main cause is infection (~60%).[9] TBSA burn, presence of inhalation injury, ventilator days, and age > 40 years are predictors of mortality

Prevention

- Pre-deployment education reduces preventable non-combat burns
- Fire-protective clothing reduces the severity of burn injuries
- Personal protective equipment may reduce penetrating injury

Specific Causes 1. Explosive Weapons

Physics

- Detonation causes an increase in pressure, which creates a blast wave or blast wind. The blast wave is high pressure travelling greater than the speed of sound. The blast wind is due to the blast wave displacing the surrounding air
- Burns arise from flashes, due to the primary effect of the explosives, or flames, due to secondary effect of explosives, eg. igniting clothing

Pathology

- Primary (barotrauma)
  - Blast wave affects air–tissue interfaces, eg. ear, lung, gastrointestinal tract. Happens within 10 metres of epicentre and is not protected by body armour[11]
- Secondary (fragmentation)
  - Penetrating trauma from surroundings. Occurs up to 1,000 metres from epicentre[12]
- Tertiary (displacement)
  - Displacement due to the blast wind causing blunt and penetrating trauma, compartment syndrome, and traumatic amputation.
- Quaternary (miscellaneous, eg. burn)
  - Affects ~25% people in an explosion[12]

Effect

- Ear. Tympanic membrane rupture. Affects ~95% therefore is a sensitive marker.[11,12] Causes transient sensorineuronal deafness (resolves in hours/days)
- Lung. From pneumothoraces to oedema and respiratory failure. Affects up to 50% of people who die.[12] Blast lung syndrome is characterized by triad of dyspnoea, bradycardia, and hypotension. Chest X-ray shows bilateral pulmonary infiltrates in a butterfly pattern but CT is more sensitive. Arterial air emboli can be seen in the retinal vessels and may cause cerebrovascular accident, myocardial infarction, and intestinal ischaemia
- Gastrointestinal. Ruptured hollow viscera secondary to haemorrhage and ischaemia
- Ocular. From conjunctival haemorrhage to ruptured globes. Affects ~10%[12]
- Musculoskeletal. Associated with traumatic amputations and mortality and therefore requires aggressive intervention. Affects ~7%[12]
- Central. From cerebral contusion to intracranial haemorrhage. 'Shell shock' encompasses concussive syndrome, post-traumatic stress disorder, and memory dysfunction

Management

- General. ATLS
- Ear. >5% rupture[10] is referred for tympanoplasty
- Lung. Oxygen. Thoracostomies are performed before anaesthetic or air transport. During ventilation high pressures are avoided to prevent air embolism and pneumothorax. Hyperbaric oxygen is considered for arterial emboli
- Gastrointestinal. Laparotomy if perforation
- Ocular. Irrigation for 60 minutes if chemical burns and specialist opinion sought
- Musculoskeletal. Gross deformity is re-aligned and fractures splinted. Surgical debridement is performed

Outcome

- Extent of injury depends upon amount and composition of material, delivery method, surrounding environment, and distance between victim and blast
- Explosions cause more polytrauma than any other wounding agent[13]
- Secondary effects of blasts are the leading cause of injury and death in military attacks[11,12]

Specific causes 2. Incendiary weapons

White phosphorous

Pathology
- Thermal and chemical burn via ignition on contact with air

Effect
- Full thickness burn with deeper extension due to high lipid solubility. Systemically causes multi-organ dysfunction

Management
- First aid via removing clothes, irrigating wound, and resuscitation with IV fluids
- Remove phosphorous particles. Ultraviolet light (Wood's lamp) is used to visualize particles. No evidence that copper sulphate aids visualization more and may cause renal failure if systemic absorption
- Excise non-viable tissue

Napalm

Pathology
- Gel mixed with petroleum that sticks to skin

Effect
- Full thickness burns with deeper extension. 10% TBSA burn can cause renal failure. Explosion can cause carbon monoxide (CO) poisoning

Management
- First aid via removing clothes, irrigating wound and resuscitation with IV fluids
- Remove napalm from skin
- If CO poisoning give 100% oxygen
- Excise non-viable tissue

Specific causes 3. Chemical weapons

Sulphur mustard gas

Pathology
- Gas or yellow-brown liquid that smells like mustard. Causes chemical burns via lipophilic action. Breaks down slowly and can damage DNA but is not usually fatal

Effect
- Produces blistering partial thickness burns with slow wound healing

Management
- Move patient to higher ground as it is heavier than air and therefore settles in low-lying areas
- First aid via removing clothes, irrigating wound, and resuscitation with IV fluids

Specific causes 4. Cold burns

Frostbite

Definitions
- Frostnip causes tissue cooling without destruction
- Frostbite causes tissue damage at temperatures below freezing point (~0.55°C)

Pathology
- At temperatures below 0°C blood vessels constrict and glomus bodies in the dermis shunt blood away from the extremities

Effect
- Symptoms include pain developing later to numbness
- Examination reveals a cold area, erythematous tissues developing later to black necrosis, blisters containing initially clear developing later to haemorrhagic fluid, and oedema

Management
- General management includes prevention (eg. protective clothing), elevation to prevent oedema, and splinting to prevent excessive movement which causes ice crystals. Rewarming is performed passively (eg. blanket) and actively (eg. whirlpool devices), and slowly for non-freezing injuries but quickly for freezing cold injuries (~40°C for 30 minutes twice daily until thawing). Frostbite is not rewarmed until the risk of refreezing is small otherwise more damage occurs[14]
- Medical management includes analgesia, antibiotics, and tetanus toxoid if necrotic tissue. Aloe vera an inhibitor of thromboxane is used for dressings every 6 hours. Thrombolysis is used if major frostbite presents <24 hours post injury and major tissue loss is predicted. Vasodilatory drug infusion, eg. Iloprost is used if major frostbite presents >24 hours post injury[14]
- Surgical debridement is performed early if complicated by infection otherwise delayed until demarcation, which may take up to ~2 months, or auto-amputation occurs. Clear blisters are debrided but not haemorrhagic ones to prevent desiccation

References

1. Jeevaratnam JA, Pandya AN. One year of burns at a role 3 medical treatment facility in Afghanistan. Journal of the Royal Army Medical Corps. 2014;160:22–6.
2. Foster MA, Moledina J, Jeffery SLA. Epidemiology of U.K. Military burns. Journal of Burn Care & Research 2011;32:415–20.
3. Wolf SE, Kauvar DS, Wade CE, Cancio LC, et al. Comparison between civilian burns and combat burns from operation Iraqi Freedom and Operation Enduring Freedom. Annals of Surgery 2006;243:786–95.
4. Page F, Hamnett N, D'Asta F, Jeffery S. Epidemiology of U.K. Military Burns 2008–2013. Journal of Burn Care Research. 2017;38(1):e269–76.
5. Roeder RA, Schulman CI. An overview of war-related thermal injuries. Journal of Craniofacial Surgery 2010;21:971–5.
6. Atiyeh BS, Hayek SN. Management of war-related burn injuries: lessons learned from recent ongoing conflicts providing exceptional care in unusual places. Journal of Craniofacial Surgery 2010;21:1529–37.
7. Chung KK, Wolf SE, Cancio LC, et al. Resuscitation of severely burned military casualties: fluid begets more fluid. Journal of Trauma 2009;67:231–7.
8. White CE, Renz EM. Advances in surgical care: management of severe burn injury. Critical Care Medicine 2008;36:S318–24.
9. Gomez R, Murray CK, Hospenthal DR, et al. Causes of mortality by autopsy findings of combat casualties and civilian patients admitted to a burns unit. Journal of the American College of Surgeons 2009;208:348–54.
10. Kauvar DS, Wolf SE, Wade CE, Cancio LC, Renz EM, Holcomb JB. Burns sustained in combat explosions in Operations Iraqui and Enduring Freedom (OIF/OEF explosion burns). Burns 2006;32:853–7.
11. Depalma RG, Burris DG, Champion HR, Hodgson MJ. Blast injuries. New England Journal of Medicine 2005;352:1335–42.
12. Wolf SJ, Bebarta VS, Bonnett CJ, et al. Blast injuries. Lancet 2009;374:405–15.
13. Champion HR, Holcomb JB, Young LA. Injuries from explosions: physics, biophysics, pathology, and required research focus. Journal of Trauma 2009;66:1468–77.
14. Hallam MJ, Cubison T, Dheansa B, Imray C. Managing frostbite. British Medical Journal 2010;341:151–6.

Sunburn and artificial tanning

Solar radiation

Radiation from the sun is electromagnetic. Most of the solar radiation is blocked by the ozone layer, dust and moisture. The solar spectrum ranges from around 230 to 3,000 nm. Visible light and infrared represent the longer wavelengths of the solar radiation spectrum. It is the shorter, ultraviolet (UV) wavelengths that are most harmful.

UV radiation

UV covers the wavelength range 100–400 nm and is divided into three bands.

UVA: 400–315 nm
- The longer wavelength penetrates further into the dermis
- Has influence at a cellular level
- Partly responsible for chronic photo-damage

UVB: 315–280 nm
- Erythematogenic
- Stimulates epidermal thickening and melanin production
- Photo-carcinogenic

UVC: 280–100 nm
- Blocked by the ozone layer
- Arises from artificial sources, eg. germicidal lamps
- Potent photo-carcinogen

Artificial tanning

- Artificial tanning is a $1 billion-a-year industry in the USA alone
- 10% of northern Europeans admitting to regular sun bed use
- This increase in sun bed use is of considerable public health concern, mainly with regard to skin cancer, but has also been in the public eye more recently as a result of burns sustained due to either ignorance or negligence on the part of the consumer or proprietor
- Sun beds predominantly emit UVA radiation, which is thought to be the least harmful UV spectrum, with varying levels of the more biologically active UVB (0.2–3.5%)
- In recent years, sun beds have been manufactured that produce higher proportions of UVB to mimic the solar spectrum and speed the tanning process
- The incidence of sun bed related burns are increasing

Acute harmful effects of UV radiation

- Pruritus
- Dryness
- Erythema
- Blistering
- Photodrug reactions
- Phototoxic/photoallergic reactions

Erythema

- Research has reported a biphasic erythema response to UVA:
  - Immediate erythema present and maximal at the end of exposure
  - Fades partly or completely
  - Followed by a later secondary phase of erythema
- The most clinically apparent component of sunburn
- Minimal erythema dose (MED) is the minimum amount of energy required to produce uniform, clearly demarcated erythema at 24 hours
- Four MED produces painful sunburn, eight MED produces blisters

Photosensitive reactions

- Term applied to abnormal reactions of human skin to UV exposure
- UVA from sun beds can produce photosensitive and phototoxic burns
- Many commonly used medications can cause phototoxic and photoallergic reactions and are activated in the UVA range
- Psoralens in many common vegetables represent a particularly dangerous substance
- UV exposure can also exacerbate photosensitive diseases such as porphyria and systemic lupus erythematosus

Management

The mainstay of treatment for sunburn is symptomatic, with regular moisturizing and pain relief. Very few patients require admission. A suggested treatment algorithm for sunburn is shown in Fig. 41.1.

Public awareness and education must play a part in preventing adverse effects of sun exposure and sun bed use. The increasing incidence of sun bed related burns highlights the need for tighter regulation of the tanning industry.

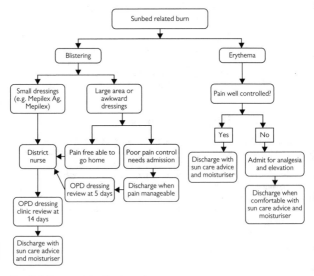

Fig. 41.1 Treatment algorithm for sunburn.

Reprinted from Hemington-Gorse SJ, et al. Burns related to sunbed use. Burns 2010;36(6):920–3, Copyright © 2010, with permission from Elsevier.

Further reading

Health & Safety Executive. Controlling the health risks from the use of UV tanning equipment. INDG209 10/95;1995.

Spencer J, Amonette R. Indoor tanning: risks, benefits, and future trends. Journal of the American Academy of Dermatology 1995;33:288–98.

World Health Organization. Artificial tanning sunbeds: risks and guidance. Geneva: WHO, 2003.

Frostbite

Definition of frostbite

Frostbite is the damage sustained by tissues when exposed to temperatures below their freezing point (<0°C).

Pattern of injury

- The severity of injury is proportional to the temperature, duration of exposure, and the depth of tissue involvement
- The spectrum of disease can vary significantly with just a small area of frostbite with minimal tissue loss, to the involvement of a whole extremity requiring amputation
- Most commonly affected extremities include: fingers, toes, nose, ears, cheeks, and genitalia

Predisposing factors

A variety of factors have been associated with the development of frostbite injury.

Extrinsic
- Prolonged exposure to cold
- Inadequate or constrictive clothing
- Extremes of age
- Military occupation
- Immobilization
- Homelessness
- Smoking
- Alcohol
- Drug abuse
- Psychiatric disease
- High altitude
- Moist/wet skin
- Afro-Caribbean descent

Intrinsic
- Dehydration and hypovolaemia
- Systemic disease: diabetes, peripheral vascular disease, Raynaud's disease
- Drugs: vasoconstrictive drugs (eg. β blockers), sedatives, neuroleptics
- Peripheral neuropathy

Clinical assessment

History

The following factors are relevant from the history to assess the severity of injury, treatment, and prognosis.

- Patient age
- Comorbidities
- Smoking status
- Drug history: medical and social
- Alcohol history
- Timing of injury
- Duration of exposure
- Temperature
- Presence of wind chill
- Periods of thawing
- Protective clothing worn
- Previous frostbite injury

Symptoms and signs

- Commonest symptoms initially are a cool extremity, sensory loss, and a feeling of clumsiness
- Frozen tissue may appear mottled blue, violaceous, yellowish-white or waxy
- Although the initial appearance of the injury may appear insignificant, the demarcation of non-viable tissue and the true extent of injury may take several weeks to determine

Classification

The severity of frostbite has been divided into four grades (Table 42.1) depending on the appearance of the extremity.

Good prognostic indicators include
- Light coloured blisters
- Normal skin colour
- Retained sensation
- Presence of oedema

Poor prognostic factors include
- Haemorrhagic blisters (indicate damage to sub-dermal vascular plexus)
- Non-blanching cyanosis
- Lack of oedema
- Firm non-deforming tissues

Table 42.1 Grading of severity of frostbite

Grade	Clinical features
First degree	**Superficial, partial thickness injury** White plaque with surrounding erythema Oedema, hyperaemia No blisters or necrosis
Second degree	**Full thickness skin freezing (dermal involvement)** Erythema, substantial oedema Vesicles with clear fluid Skin desquamation and formation of black eschar
Third degree	**Full thickness skin and subcutaneous freezing** Haemorrhagic blisters Skin necrosis Blue-grey discolouration
Fourth degree	**Full thickness necrosis** Involving skin, subcutaneous tissue, muscle, tendon and bone Minimal oedema Initially mottling, deep red or cyanotic In late stages, dry, black and mummified

Pathophysiology

Local cold injury produces a series of progressive, overlapping changes that are divided into
1. Pre-freeze phase
2. Freeze thaw phase
3. Vascular stasis phase
4. Late ischaemic phase

The injury associated with frostbite occurs by two mechanisms.
1. Direct cell damage and death from cold injury
2. Vascular changes leading to progressive tissue ischaemia

Cellular injury

- Cellular injury occurs through the formation of ice crystals
- When freezing is gradual, ice crystals initially form in the extracellular space, increasing the extracellular osmotic pressure. This draws water across the cell membrane leading to intracellular dehydration and altered cell haemostasis due to electrolyte and pH imbalance
- With continued freezing, there is formation of intracellular ice crystals, enzyme destruction, decreased DNA synthesis, and a localized vascular response due to release of histamine from the injured cell
- In contrast, if the freezing is very rapid, intracellular ice crystals are formed prior to extracellular crystals, leading to more severe cell damage and death

Vascular changes

The triad of vasoconstriction, endothelial injury and thromboembolism contribute to the vascular insufficiency and tissue ischaemia seen in frostbite.
- Freezing leads to vasoconstriction which leads to reduced blood flow and exacerbates skin cooling to produce further vasoconstriction
- Cooling of vascular contents leads to loss of the vascular endothelial integrity, which precipitates fibrin deposition, transcapillary plasma loss, and oedema formation. Oedema formation is further exacerbated by mast cell degranulation and histamine release from the damaged endothelial cells
- Cooling and endothelial damage also results in increased blood viscosity and vascular stasis with formation of microemboli that occlude capillaries

Inflammatory response

- The progressive changes and inflammatory response observed in frostbite injury is similar to that of a burn wound
- Freezing leads to the release of pro-inflammatory mediators with high levels of prostaglandin $F_{2\alpha}$ ($PGF_{2\alpha}$) and thromboxane$_{A2}$ (TXA_2) detected in frostbite blisters. These factors have been implicated in vasoconstriction, platelet aggregation, and leucocyte adhesion which worsen the ischaemia

Freeze–thaw–refreeze cycles

- The 'freeze–thaw–refreeze' cycles are thought to produce the most damage than the initial ice crystal formation in the tissues
- Refreezing after thawing produces intracellular ice crystal formation with extensive cell destruction and further release of prothrombotic and vasoconstrictive $PGF_{2\alpha}$ and TXA_2 which in turn cause progressive thrombosis and ischaemia

Imaging

Imaging can help determine the severity and depth of injury. A variety of modalities have been used including plain radiographs, laser Doppler studies, digital plethysmography, infrared thermography, and MRI. Triple phase bone scanning (technitium-99) and MRI are the most useful adjuncts to clinical practice.

- Plain radiographs can demonstrate soft-tissue swelling initially. With time, tissue loss, bone demineralization, and periosteal inflammation can be evident
- Technetium scans can be useful in the first few days after injury to determine the extent of tissue necrosis to allow for early debridement and coverage of bony structures. However, technetium scintigraphy fails to show the condition of the surrounding tissues or demarcate the level of soft-tissue ischaemia
- MRI is regarded as a more superior modality as it allows direct visualization of the occluded vessels, images the adjacent tissues, and clearly demarcates the ischaemic tissues, which can aid surgical planning prior to debridement

Treatment

General management
- Patients with significant frostbite injury should be admitted to a specialist unit
- Potentially life-threatening conditions, eg. hypothermia (core body temperature <35°C) and concomitant injuries take priority over frostbite injuries
- A core temperature of 34°C should be achieved prior to rewarming of the affected extremity
- Intravenous fluid resuscitation is only indicated if the patient is dehydrated or has concomitant injuries

Rewarming
- The initial treatment of frostbite should follow the protocol outlined by McCauley, Heggers, and Robson.[1]
- Rewarming should be carried out in a whirlpool bath of recirculating water containing a mild antiseptic (povo-iodine or chlorhexidine) set at a temperature of 40–41°C
- Rewarming should continue for at least 30 minutes or until thawing is complete and the tissues are pliable and red-purple in colour.
- The treatment is repeated twice daily for 30 minutes until there is clear demarcation of necrotic tissues or until healing is observed
- The affected area is kept dry and warm in between the treatments

Supportive treatments
- Adequate analgesia with an opiate should be administered; intense pain is experienced 2–3 days after rewarming and reperfusion, which may persist for weeks even after demarcation of tissues
- Ibuprofen should be given (400 mg every 12 hours) as it has anti-prostaglandin effects
- Once the extremity has thawed, clear blisters should be de-roofed while haemorrhagic blisters should be kept intact
- Avoid massage/rubbing to the affected area as it can cause further damage
- Topical aloe vera has been used in North America on wounds after blister debridement due to its anti-prostaglandin effects
- Affected extremities should be elevated as extracellular crystals melt with rewarming, causing hyperaemia and oedema
- Broad-spectrum prophylactic antibiotics are indicated if there is a risk of infection from necrotic tissue

Treatment of frostbite
- Admit to a specialized unit
- Treat hypothermia or life threatening concomitant injuries first
- Remove wet or constrictive clothing
- Rewarm with a warm water bath (40–41°C) for at least 30 minutes or until thawing
- Repeat treatment twice daily for 30 minutes
- Keep the extremity warm and dry in between rewarming sessions
- After rewarming, debride clear blisters
- Leave haemorrhagic blisters
- Elevate the extremity and splint as necessary
- Avoid smoking
- Administer ibuprofen (400 mg every 12 hours orally)
- Anti-tetanus prophylaxis
- Opiate analgesia
- Broad spectrum antibiotics if there is a risk of infection from necrotic tissues
- Clear documentation with photos taken every 2–3 days is essential
- Avoid massage/rubbing or direct heat to the affected area

Surgery
- Tissue may become viable for rewarming despite their initial appearance and demarcation of non-viable tissues can take weeks
- Early surgical intervention is therefore only indicated for
  - Compartment syndrome or vascular impairment requiring a fasciotomy or escharotomy
  - Gross sepsis, liquefaction or gangrene, requiring amputation of the extremity
- Tissue loss is uncommon in first- and second-degree frostbite injuries
- In third- and fourth-degree injuries, once the necrotic tissues has demarcated, mummification and auto-amputation may be allowed to occur or surgical debridement with amputation or reconstruction can be performed (Fig. 42.1)

Tissue plasminogen activator
- Tissue plasminogen activator (tPA) can lead to rapid clearance of vascular thromboses, restore arterial perfusion, and improve tissue salvage
- Significant reduction in digital amputation rates have been demonstrated with tPA
- tPA therapy should be considered in patients with severe extremity frostbite presenting within 24 hours of the injury
- Diagnostic angiography can used to guide treatment and tPA therapy should be repeated until reperfusion is confirmed on the angiogram
- Therapy is contraindicated in cases of concomitant trauma, recent surgery, bleeding diasthesis, pregnancy, repeated freeze–thaw cycles, or neurological impairment

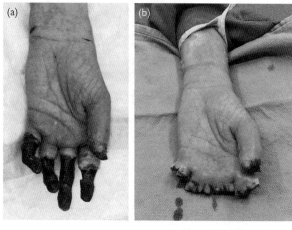

Fig. 42.1 Severe frostbite requiring subtotal digital amputation. (A) before and (B) after amputation.

Vasodilators
- Some benefit demonstrated but their role has not been fully substantiated
- Examples include iloprost (prostacyclin analogue), buflomedil (α-blocker), and pentoxifylline (a methyl-xanthine derived phosphodiesterase)

Sympathectomy
- May help to reduce oedema, decrease tissue loss, and prevent long-term sequelae, eg. pain and paraesthesia
- Chemical or surgical sympathectomy, performed 24–48 hours after thawing has demonstrated equivocal results

Hyperbaric oxygen
- Safe and inexpensive treatment
- It increases the deformability of erythrocytes, reduces tissue oedema, and has antioxidant and has antibacterial effects
- Benefit of hyperbaric oxygen with large human studies has yet to be determined

Long-term sequelae

- Hypersensitivity to cold
- Sensory deficits
- Chronic pain
- Hyperhidrosis
- Heterotropic calcification
- Pigmentary changes
- Osteoporosis
- Subchondral bone loss
- Growth plate abnormalities in children
- Susceptibility to further frostbite injury

Prevention

Prevention is key and a variety of protective measures can help reduced the occurrence of frostbite injuries.
- Avoid prolonged cold exposure
- Protective clothing worn—multiple loose layers for heat insulation
- Wear insulated or heated insoles, gloves, and hats
- Avoid constrictive or tight clothing that reduce blood flow
- Take protection from the wind
- Keep extremities dry
- Avoid smoking and alcohol
- Maintain nutrition and hydration
- Supplementary oxygen at high altitudes

Further reading

Hallam MJ, Cubison T, Dheansa B, Imray C. Managing frostbite. British Medical Journal 2010;341:1151–6.
Murphy JV, Banwell PE, Roberts AHN, McGrouther DA. Frostbite: pathogenesis and treatment. Journal of Trauma 2000;48:171–8.

References

1. McCauley RL, Heggers JP, Robson MC. Frostbite. Methods to minimize tissue loss. Postgrad Med. 1990;88(8):67–8, 73–7.

Hair restoration

Introduction to hair restoration

Scalp and facial hair are essential components of what is perceived to be normal appearance. Hair regrowth after a burn injury is often as much a concern for the patient as scar disfigurement. Surgical hair restoration should be delayed until the patient is fully recovered from the acute phase of the burn injury.

A description of the anatomy and physiology of the hair follicle is beyond the scope of this chapter but it is important to have an understanding of this when considering hair restoration surgery.

Options for management

Not all patients will be suitable for surgery and the burn multi-disciplinary team should be aware of the non-surgical choices available to the patient. These include:

• Cosmetic camouflage—scalp dyes, microfiber sprays, eyebrow make-up
• Semi-permanent micro-pigmentation
• Scalp hair restoration systems – partial hair pieces or complete wigs
• Hair-bearing adhesive prostheses—eyebrows, false eyelashes
• Scalp hair bearing prostheses combined with Branemark ear prostheses

The surgical options will depend on the location of the hair bearing area affected and the size of the defect (Table 43.1). These include:

• Serial excision with or without tissue expansion
• Hair-bearing flaps with or without tissue expansion
• Hair-bearing full thickness grafts
• Hair transplantation

In male patients where hair-bearing flaps are being considered, it is important to understand the potential for male pattern hair loss in the future and warn the patient that flaps taken from areas that are genetically predetermined to lose hair will do so in their transferred location which may lead to unnatural patterns of balding. In some cases such loss can be prevented by using approved medications for androgenetic alopecia such as oral finasteride or topical minoxidil.

Hair transplantation for scalp scars should be considered as an option provided that the donor to recipient area ratio is appropriate. Donor hair harvesting can be maximized using the traditional occipital strip (Fig 43.1) but in selected cases follicular unit excision may be considered. Both techniques produce grafts (see Fig. 43.1) that are implanted into multiple incisions. Results that can be achieved are shown in Fig. 43.2

Even if flaps or serial excisions are utilized, hair transplants can be used to refine hairlines and sideburns, and fill in non hair-bearing surgical scars (Fig. 43.3).

Table 43.1 Scalp burn scar alopecia classification

Type I	Single alopecia segment
	A Less than 25% of the hair-bearing scalp
	B 20–50% of the hair-bearing scalp
	C 50–75% of the hair-bearing scalp
	D 75% of the hair-bearing scalp
Type II	Multiple alopecia segments amenable to tissue expansion
Type III	Patchy burn alopecia not amenable to tissue expansion
Type IV	Total alopecia

Reproduced from McCauley RL et al., Tissue expansion in the correction of burn alopecia: classification and methods of correction. Annals of Plastic Surgery 25(2):103–15, Copyright © 1990, with permission from Lippincott Williams & Wilkins.

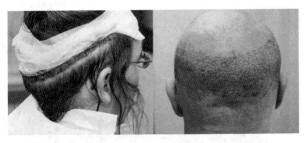

Fig. 43.1 Donor hair harvesting methods–Strip Follicular Unit Transplantation (Strip FUT) vs Follicular Unit Excision (FUE).

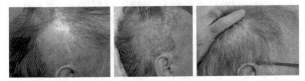

Fig. 43.2 Results of hair transplant surgery.

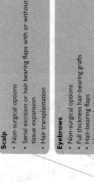

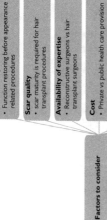

Scalp
- Non-surgical options
- Serial excision or hair bearing flaps with or without tissue expansion
- Hair transplantation

Eyebrows
- Non-surgical options
- Full thickness hair-bearing grafts
- Hair-bearing flaps
- Hair transplantation

Eyelashes
- Non-surgical options
- Hair transplantation- gandelman technique or direct implantation

Moustache, beard and sideburns
- Non-surgical options
- Serial excision with or without tissue expansion
- Hair transplantation

Other areas including Chest, limbs, axillae and pubic region –
- Serial excision with or without tissue expansion
- Hair transplantation

Factors to consider

Problem list prioritisation
- Function restoring before appearance related procedures

Scar quality
- scar maturity is required for hair transplant procedures

Availability of expertise
- Reconstructive surgeons vs hair transplant surgeons

Cost
- Private vs public health care provision

General health and nutritional status
- Vitamin/trace element and hormonal/endocrine imbalances can affect hair growth

Patient expectation
- E.g. tissue expansion commitment vs hair transplant delay to see result

Anatomical area involved in burn scar

Age
- Children may not be suitable for hair transplant procedures because of lack of compliance

Gender
- Awareness in males of the potential for male pattern hair loss including family history

Fig. 43.3 Factors to consider when planning hair restoration in burn scars.

Conclusion

Hair restoration in burn scars is a specialized field with a number of options that may not all be available locally within the burns centre. It is important for the multidisciplinary team to be aware of the possible therapeutic modalities and to develop established links with practitioners who offer those services that are not available locally. Consultations should be co-ordinated and streamlined so that the treatment options are discussed with the patients prior to their making an informed decision on management of post burn alopecia.

Further reading

Farjo B, Farjo N, Williams G. Hair transplantation in burn scar alopecia. Scars, Burns & Healing 2015;12059513115607764.

Laser management of scars

Introduction to laser management of scars

There is increasing interest and evidence that laser therapy can help in the management of scars. Owing to accessibility, variations in education and training, cost of lasers, and disparate nature of scars there is still much work to be done in relation to indications and outcomes.

Potential therapeutic interventions with lasers for scars

Erythema

The pulsed dye laser at 585–595 nm has potentially the greatest evidence base for scar treatment, especially in hypertrophic scars. It is the most effective laser for reducing erythema. Some reports of success with deeper vascularity with Nd:YAG laser have been published.

Hair bearing skin

Depending on skin type, the alexandrite or Nd:YAG lasers and some diode lasers are the most useful for depilation in the context of burn-related folliculitis.

Pigmentation

Q-switched Nd:YAG and ablative lasers, such as the carbon dioxide laser, can help with areas of hyperpigmentation. Patient selection based on skin type is important to avoid complications such as worsening the problem or hypopigmentation. Some benefit has also been reported from intense pulsed light (IPL).

Hypopigmentation

Hypopigmentation may occur in all skin types following thermal injury, but is more prevalent in the higher Fitzpatrick scale skin types. This is a very difficult problem to treat and the role of lasers remains unclear, but there is potential promise in laser resurfacing combined with autologous keratinocytes, although this remains a matter for further research.

Hypertrophic and keloid scarring

Hypertrophic and keloid scarring responds to vascular lasers such as pulsed dye laser (PDL) or long pulsed Nd:Yag laser with variable but often good results. It may be beneficial to concurrently treat established keloid scarring with intralesional steroid injections and persisting with less invasive treatments such as pressure garments. It is well established that PDL treatment in keloid scarring can lead to improved density and texture as well as reduced irritation and pruritus in addition to reducing overall scar volume. Fractional or totally ablative laser resurfacing with the CO_2 laser can be of considerable benefit, but results can be unpredictable and treatment should be undertaken in the context of multimodal therapy.

Inconsistencies in texture

Scar resurfacing, following grafting or aberrant natural healing processes, may be achieved with fractionated carbon dioxide laser. All ablative treatments must take into consideration the thickness and quality of the skin being treated and the density of pilo-sebaceous units: skin grafts will respond differently to native skin. Some benefit has also been achieved with erbium:YAG fractional resurfacing.

Post-procedural considerations

Re-epithelialization after laser treatment relies upon the mobilization of epidermal cells from the pilosebaceous units; areas that have fewer units or where the units are significantly damaged may be slower to heal. Patients with higher Fitzpatrick scale skin type scores will be more susceptible to side effects of laser treatment and may therefore require longer treatment courses at a lower fluence. A risk–benefit analysis should be undertaken in every case, bearing the side effect profile, Fitzpatrick skin type, and predictability of response in mind.

Potential side effects of ablative laser therapy

- Immediate skin whitening
- Pain
- Infection
- Erythema, purpura
- Oedema
- Blistering, serous discharge
- Delayed wound healing
- Discolouration
- Textural change
- Hyperpigmentation

While non-ablative therapies are not without risk, the chances of side effects are greatly reduced. A test patch should be undertaken before laser treatment to minimize risk and maximize benefit.

Summary

Laser treatment is gradually establishing a firm footing as mainstream in the battle against scars. A tailored treatment programme and clear communication are of utmost importance in delivering a high-quality laser service. In order to offer a comprehensive laser scar service, a variety of ablative and non-ablative laser modalities with highly trained staff is required, preferably incorporated within a multi-modality multidisciplinary team offering a wide spectrum of scar interventions and psychological input. Owing to the expense of lasers and the high level of experience and training required, treatment is best delivered in centres of focused expertise in association with a burns unit.

Further reading

Shokrollahi K (ed.). Laser management of scars. Springer-Nature. 2019.

McGoldrick RB, Sawyer A, Davis CR, et al. Lasers and ancillary treatment for scar management: persona experience over two decades and contextual review of the literature. Part 1: Burn scars. Scars, Burns & Healing 2:2059513116642090.

McGoldrick, RB, Theodorakopoulou, E, Azzopardi, E. Lasers and ancillary treatments for scar management Part 2: Keloid, hypertrophic, pigmented and acne scars. Scars, Burns & Healing 2017;3:205951311689805.

Face transplantation

Introduction to face transplantation

Facial composite tissue allotransplantation (CTA) refers to the en bloc transplantation of hard and soft facial tissue between two non-related persons. In severe cases of facial disfigurement, as may occur following burn injury, facial CTA has the potential to restore aesthetic and functional derangements beyond that which conventional reconstructive options currently allow. This benefit must be weighed against the need for lifelong immunosuppression and risk of rejection. In the properly selected patient, however, facial CTA can be a transformative operation.

History of face transplantation

- First face transplant performed in 2005 in Amiens, France
- Total of 22 partial or full facial transplantations have been performed worldwide to date
- Five of these patients have medium-term follow-up
- All have experienced acute rejection episodes; no reported commensurate loss of transplant
- One patient died of unclear cause, another died secondary to severe infection (face and hand transplantation)

Patient indications for face transplantation

Patients recovering from burn injuries in the face may have significant aesthetic and functional concerns secondary to excessive facial scarring and contracture. Indications for facial transplantation in the burn patient are similar to those having suffered major facial trauma and include:

- Severe disfigurement, usually encompassing soft tissue loss more than 25% of facial surface area
- Loss of multiple facial units considered difficult to reconstruct, including nose, eyelids, and lips
- Loss of multiple facial functions, including eating, drinking, speaking, breathing through the nose, and the ability for facial expression
- Multiple reconstructive facial operations performed without satisfactory aesthetic or functional outcome
- Indications for the procedure are ever changing and contingent upon advancements in immunosuppressive medication, synthetic materials, and expanding reconstructive options

Patient selection

Following facial CTA, patients engage actively in rehabilitation during the first few years postoperatively to assist in the process of regaining facial function. Furthermore, patients must remain accessible, as their care requires frequent and involved medical surveillance, including scheduled biopsies and laboratory tests and urgent assessments of potential episodes of rejection or opportunistic infection. Therefore, patients must be otherwise physically and mentally healthy to participate in and gain benefit from the procedure.

- Patients must not have a recent history of malignancies, chronic infections which may be potentiated by immunosuppression, or other significant chronic diseases which may be life-threatening or limiting
- Psychiatrist screening necessary to diagnose existing psychological disorders
- Must assess history of alcohol and substance abuse, as well as social support
- Determine and plan for logistical issues in maintaining frequent follow-up
- Use of human allograft skin and blood transfusion during the acute burn care seems to lead to high level of pre-sensitization; possibly limiting donor selection

Outcomes of facial composite tissue allotransplantation

Medical outcomes

- Complications reported in the acute postoperative phase include infections, hematoma, and lymphadenopathy
- Patients enrolled in our immunosuppression protocol have suffered, at most, one episode of acute rejection
- Opportunistic infections have occurred in three patients
- Metabolic and haematologic complications include new onset diabetes, steroid-induced confusion, haemolytic anaemia, hypertension, and acute renal failure
- No evidence for new neoplastic growth

Functional outcomes

- All patients demonstrate progressively improving 2-point discrimination
- Return of sensation to transplanted segment in 3–6 months, slower return of facial expression
- Facial expression slower to return than sensory and varies in degree of success. There may be asymmetry between each side of the face
- All patients able to achieve some level of autonomous oral feeding within first 2 weeks
- Normal food bolus mobilization slower to return
- Speech correlates with success of facial reanimation

Social outcomes

- All patients self-report dramatic improvement in post-transplantation appearance
- All report increase in self-esteem and self-appearance

Summary

Facial CTA offers an alternative approach to extensive facial injuries, which may be otherwise very difficult to restore. Although there are significant risks associated with the procedure, it can be a powerful reconstructive tool to restore both facial form and function in the carefully selected patient. Additionally, human skin allografts should be used cautiously in treatment of acute burn patients as they limit a possible match of donors, while acceptable alternative dressings exist (Fig. 45.1).

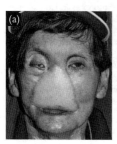 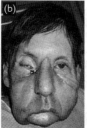 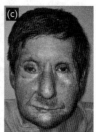

Fig. 45.1 The figure demonstrates the operative course of a patient who suffered a 4th degree electrical burn of the face, including loss of nose, maxilla, and upper lip. Preoperatively (A), the patient has a flap covering his midface defect following extensive debridement. (B) Acute postoperative period. (B) The patient is within the acute period following facial CTA. (C) The patient has undergone minor revisions.

Figure 45.1A reproduced with permission from Pomahac B et al. Restoration of facial form and function after severe disfigurement from burn injury by a composite facial allograft. American Journal of Transplantation 201;11(2):386–93, Copyright © 2011 The Authors. Journal Compilation, Copyright © 2011 The American Society of Transplantation and the American Society of Transplant Surgeons.

Further reading

Barret JP, Gavaldà J, Bueno J, et al. Full face transplant: the first case report. Annals of Surgery 2011;254:252–6.

Cendales LC, Kanitakis J, Schneeberger S, et al. The Banff 2007 working classification of skin-containing composite tissue allograft pathology. American Journal of Transplantation 2008;8:1396–400.

Dubernard JM, Lengelé B, Morelon E, et al. Outcomes 18 months after the first human partial face transplantation. New England Journal of Medicine 2007;357:2451–60.

Fischer S, Kueckelhaus M, Pauzenberger R, et al. Functional outcomes of face transplantation. American Journal of Transplantation 2015;15:220–33.

National Geographic. The Story of a Face. September 2018.

Petruzzo P, Lanzetta M, Dubernard JM, et al. The International Registry on Hand and Composite Tissue Transplantation. Transplantation 2010;90:1590–4.

Pomahac B, Nowinski D, Diaz-Siso JR, et al. Face transplantation. Current Problems in Surgery 2011;48:293–357.

Theodorakopoulou, E, Meghji, S, Pafitanis, G. A review of the world's published face transplant cases: ethical perspectives. Scars, Burns & Healing 2017;3: 1–10. Doi: 10.1177/2059513117694402.

Pain management

Introduction to pain management

Treatment of pain in the burn patient presents a unique set of challenges. The pathology of pain with these injuries, while consistent at its most basic level, varies considerably with factors such as the burn severity and the stage of treatment/healing. The experience of pain shows similar variation. The assessment of pain and recognition of contributing factors such as anxiety and depression require vigilance and persistence, especially among paediatric populations. A systematic approach to pain management can help to ensure adequate, consistent treatment of pain and may be implemented in the form of a pain protocol. We recommend that the adult/paediatric British National Formulary is used to ensure correct doses are given when not known.

Pathophysiology

Initial injury

Noxious thermal stimuli are transduced by peripheral nociceptors in the skin and their signals are relayed via A and C nerve fibres to the central nervous system. Modulation of the sensitivity of these fibres may play a role in the development of the hyperalgesia that is commonly seen in burn wounds and surrounding tissues. The pattern of pain, but not necessarily its intensity, following this initial stimulus is dependent upon the severity of the burn injury.

- Superficial partial thickness burns typically produce mild pain that is especially aggravated by frictional stimuli such as clothing
- Deep partial thickness burns produce pain that varies in intensity according to the extent of dermal destruction. Burns extending only to the superficial dermis produce the most painful injuries, leaving the nerve endings of the dermis stripped of the protective epidermis
- Full thickness burns may be insensate to sharp stimulus, at least initially. Still, these deeper burns may be associated with a dull or pressure-like pain that worsens as the inflammatory process progresses

Treatment/healing period

Despite the overall trend of pain decreasing with time, there exists considerable variation in pain reports. This variation is partly attributed to the increases in pain associated with surgical procedures and other wound therapies.

- For the purposes of assessment and treatment, categorizing pain as procedural or background is useful
- As deeper, previously anaesthetic wounds heal, granulation tissue brings new nerve endings to life and the return of sharp pain sensation
- During this time, the potential exists for the development of chronic pain syndromes such as complex regional pain syndrome and phantom limb pain
- Providers must also be vigilant for psychological factors contributing to pain, including depression and anxiety, and address them

Assessment of pain

Multiple techniques for the measurement of pain in patients have been evaluated and are suitable for routine use.

- These include numeric scales, agitation scales, and visual analogue scales
- Assessment of pain in paediatric patients poses challenges. For pre-school and school-aged children, self-reporting of pain levels is possible, and tools tailored to each age group have been developed. For non-verbal children, other techniques can be employed such as behaviour and observation scales

More important than the technique used is the frequent and consistent application to guide and evaluate therapy.

Treatment strategies

General aspects

- A multimodal approach to the treatment of pain should be employed.
- Any therapy should be tailored to the individual patient's stage of treatment and be guided by systematic and frequent assessments and monitoring
- Pain specialist consultation should be considered early on.
- Organ dysfunctions such as renal or respiratory failure have to be taken into account regarding any pain management plan.
- Protocols should be implemented to treat pain and pain management-associated side effects such as pruritus, constipation, nausea, and vomiting, or respiratory depression
- During the resuscitative phase after a burn, intravenous (IV) analgesics should be chosen due to the potentially altered pharmacokinetics of intramuscular (IM), or per oral (PO) routes of administration.
- Opioid analgesics are the mainstay during the resuscitative phase with patient-controlled analgesia (PCA) a preferred mode of delivery in adult and select paediatric groups
- Treat pain actively to avoid breakthrough pain; scheduled preferred over as-needed administration if no side effects
- After the resuscitative phase, background pain has to be separated from procedural pain (or pain related to activity such as physical therapy); analgesics should be adjusted
- With the frequent concomitant need for sedation during procedures, medications with both analgesic and sedative properties have particular utility (ketamine)
- Consider transitioning to PO analgesics when condition stabilizes and PO absorption becomes more predictable.
- Regional analgesia can be considered if deemed appropriate; the anaesthesiology service should be consulted

Pharmacological therapies

Opioid analgesics

Opioid analgesics act on specific receptors in the central nervous system, but also in the periphery.

- Opiate analgesics form the mainstay of therapy, especially during the initial phase
- Flexibility in the route of administration: PO, IV, subcutaneous (SC), IM, rectal, intranasal, transmucosal, transdermal, and neuraxial
- Includes morphine, hydromorphone, fentanyl, pethidine, and methadone
- Opioids are equianalgesics if dose and route of administration, as well as incomplete cross-tolerance and variation in the patient's response, are considered
- Opioids have a similar profile of side effects:
  • Respiratory and cardiovascular depression, sedation, euphoria, dysphoria, nausea, vomiting, constipation, and pruritus
  • If opioids are considered, a prophylaxis against constipation should be initiated

- Specific antagonists are available (eg. naloxone) to reverse life-threatening side effects, but also will reverse the analgesic response
- May be associated with the development of tolerance, physical dependence, addiction, and pseudoaddiction. However, these concerns should not limit the use if indicated
- Tolerance and hyperalgesia has been observed, especially in ventilated patients, leading to poorly controlled pain. Adjuvants such as ketamine or clonidine have been used successfully in these critical situations
- Special legal requirements and documentation must be followed

Morphine
- Standard opioid analgesic. Metabolites can accumulate in renal failure

Fentanyl
- Eighty times more potent than morphine, rapid onset, metabolites inactive

Remifentanil
- Potent with rapid onset, but also ultrashort duration of action requires continuous infusion. Useful for procedural pain

Pethidine
- Possesses some local anaesthetic activity as well. It can be used to treat postoperative shivering. Metabolites can accumulate in renal failure, causing central nervous system excitement and resultant seizures

Methadone
- Longer half-life gives smoother control and it is effective when pain is poorly controlled by morphine due to tolerance, opioid induced hyperalgesia, or neuropathic pain

Opioid analgesics: patient-controlled analgesia (PCA)
Allows the patient to titrate his opioid medication (usually IV) via a pump, to effect and provides more patient autonomy. Only the patient is to use the PCA demand button.
- Morphine, fentanyl, hydromorphone, and pethidine are commonly used, with none being particularly superior
- Patients may need a loading dose of an opioid analgesic before initiation of PCA
- The use of a continuous opioid infusion in addition to demand dosing may be considered when variability in plasma opioid levels is leading to severe breakthrough pain. Special monitoring should be instituted, however, to monitor for drug overdose
- PCA requires special equipment and operator failure is a risk factor

Ketamine
- Depending on the dose, it has analgesic and hypnotic effects. Its NMDA receptor antagonism may be useful in cases of opiate tolerance and neuropathic pain
- It contrasts with opioids in its preservation of respiratory drive
- Associated dysphoria can be an issue in adolescents and adults which can be effectively prevented/treated with benzodiazepines

Clonidine
- It is an α2 adrenergic agonist-possessing analgesic has sedative properties
- Has opiate-sparing effects when used during procedures
- Its main side effects include sedation and hypotension, which may limit use during the acute phase after burn in critically ill patients
- Rebound hypertension may occur with abrupt discontinuation of clonidine but only in cases of chronic use

Non-steroidal anti-inflammatory drugs (NSAIDs)
- Their use in the acute phase is limited due to a side effect profile that includes platelet inhibition, renal dysfunction, and gastrointestinal complications
- They do reduce the classic metabolic response to burn injury.
- NSAIDs are useful adjuncts to opioid medications and an opioid-sparing effect has been noted

Paracetamol/acetaminophen
- It possesses opiate-sparing properties with minimal side effects when compared to NSAIDs
- Daily intake should be limited to avoid hepatic toxicity and special care should be taken when other paracetamol-containing medications, such as various oral hydrocodone preparations, are given

Topicals
- The use of topically applied analgesics, including local anaesthetics, NSAIDs, opioids, and ketamine, has been evaluated with limited success
- Topical lidocaine shows benefit but is limited by the burn size due to systemic absorption and associated toxicity

Adjuvants for neuropathic pain, burn-induced pruritus, anxiety
Gabapentin
- Gabapentin can be used in patients with neuropathic pain and patients with burn wound-induced pruritus
- It can accumulate in renal failure and renal dosing guidelines should be followed
- Its main side effects are sedation and peripheral oedema. It should not be discontinued abruptly
- Pregabalin (Lyrica) is an alternative for patients refractory/intolerant to gabapentin and similar caution should be exercised in patients with renal failure
- Dosing and safety has not been established in paediatric patients

Tricyclic antidepressants
- Oral preparations such as amitriptyline or nortriptyline show efficacy in the treatment of neuropathic pain. These medications may take a considered amount of time before an effect is noted
- Topical preparations of doxepin can be used to treat pruritus, although its use may be limited by excess sedation

Antihistamines
- Useful in treatment of anxiety and burn-induced pruritus
- Main side effect: sedation

Benzodiazepines
- Potent anxiolytics with apparent opioid-sparing properties in cases where anxiety is contributing to pain
- Useful as procedural premedication
- Added benefit of muscle relaxation, especially diazepam

Surgical therapies
- Closure of open wounds can markedly reduce pain levels.
- For full-thickness burns, early excision and grafting, if possible, is ideal
- Use of temporary measures such as xenograft, allograft, or synthetic dressings, like biobrane, is extremely beneficial for pain control as well, especially for second-degree burns

Non-pharmacological and psychological therapies
- Given that pain is complex in nature, with strong contributions from psychological factors, a multimodal approach to pain management should address these factors as well
- This includes a psychologist/psychiatrist
- As mentioned before, anxiety and depression can exacerbate pain and should be treated when identified
- Active efforts to prevent such negative psychological consequences should be employed by using strategies based on cognitive approaches as well as operant and classical conditioning
- Cognitive techniques can involve improving patients' coping by giving them more control over their treatment, especially procedures. They can be guided in restructuring their thoughts on pain to more constructive ones
- Distraction is an additional technique that follows under this category and one that technology is bringing to the forefront via virtual reality
- Operant conditioning requires addressing how caregivers respond to patient pain behaviours. Patients are rewarded for constructive behaviour such as meeting therapy goals. Reinforcement of negative behaviours such as avoidance of therapy and drug seeking are strictly avoided
- A classical conditioning approach can be implemented by thoroughly preparing patients for what to expect during procedures/therapies and making the whole experience as non-threatening as possible
- Support groups

Further reading

Allman K, Wilson I, O'Donnell A. Oxford handbook of anaesthesia. Oxford: Oxford University Press, 2011.

Meyer WJ, Martyn JA, Wiechman S, et al. Total Burn Care, 5th. Edinburgh: Elsevier, 2018; pp. 679–99.

Chapter 47

Burn care drug formulary

Analgesia

Overview

Many factors affect the most appropriate choice of analgesic agent. It is worth first considering the following factors.

- How big is the burn area?
- Is the burn mainly full thickness or partial thickness in nature?
- Has any of the uninjured skin area been used for grafts?
- Is the patient sedated or awake and alert?
- Is the patient ventilated and if so what type of ventilation (full support of respiratory effort through to continuous positive airways pressure delivered via a tracheostomy)?
- Are we aiming to treat background pain with this therapy or incident pain caused by dressings changes or physiotherapy?
- Consider using an objective measure or validated pain score (such as the short form McGill pain score or the abbreviated Burn-Specific Pain Anxiety Scale) to assess therapy failure/success
- What route do we want to use including changing routes as the patient improves (eg. switching iv to oral)?
- Do we require an analgesic weaning regimen?

Also remember to consider the following

- Simple analgesia given regularly if not contraindicated can be very effective, especially when used in conjunction with other agents of a different class. For example paracetamol 1 g qds regularly (orally or intravenously) should be considered in all patients
- Non-steroidal anti-inflammatory agents (NSAIDs) should be used with extreme caution especially in patients with bigger burns and those on intensive care in whom the risk of gastrointestinal haemorrhage and acute kidney injury is greater than that in the normal population
- When prescribing opioids also consider starting a stimulant or softening laxative such as senna 15 mg night or docusate sodium 200 mg twice daily to prevent constipation
- Take in to account and continue where possible any analgesics the patient is already on at home. For example if the patient already takes 100 mg daily of oral morphine, doses of 2.5 mg intravenously for incident pain such as dressings changes are likely to be insufficient
- If the patient is awake and alert a PCA (patient-controlled analgesia) system may be appropriate
- Burns patients may have multiple types of pain, for example in an explosion in addition to the burn a patient may also have sustained bone fractures, etc.

Opioid analgesics

- Opioids are the most common choice of analgesic
- They are easy to deliver
- come in many presentations (IV, oral, etc.) and formulations (immediate release, modified release)
- Doctors and nurses are familiar with most of them
- The common agents are relatively cheap

Morphine

Advantages

- Available in many different forms and formulations. For example intravenous injection, oral (slow release, immediate release, etc.)
- Cheap
- Effective
- can be used intravenously

Disadvantages

- May accumulate over time especially in patients with renal dysfunction, although morphine is hepatically metabolized morphine-6-glucuronide, one of the main metabolites, is active, a potent analgesic, and renally excreted so will accumulate in renal dysfunction
- Causes histamine release and therefore may precipitate anaphylactoid reactions

Fentanyl

- Synthetic opioid with an analgesic potency of approximately 50–80 times that of morphine

Advantages

- Can be given in the critical care setting as a continuous infusion in patients with renal impairment. Hepatically metabolized, metabolites have no significant analgesic active
- Minimal histamine release
- Many immediate release preparations with novel routes of administration for patient with difficult to manage incident pain. For example intranasal sprays, buccal, and sublingual tablets
- Topical patches may be of use in stable pain (25 μg/h fentanyl patch is approximately equivalent to 60–90 mg/day of oral morphine and therefore 30–45 mg of intravenous morphine) but caution is required in the placement of the patch. For example, avoid unhealed donor site

Disadvantages

- Large volume of distribution so will accumulate over time when given as a continuous infusion
- Potent respiratory depressant (this may be an advantage in some circumstances)
- May cause chest wall rigidity

Alfentanil

- Synthetic opioid with an analgesic potency of approximately 10–20 times that of morphine

- Nasal/buccal spray available in the UK through specials manufacturer which may be of use in patients with difficult to manage/control incident pain; quicker onset of action than oral morphine

Advantages
- Can be given in the critical care setting as a continuous infusion in patients with renal impairment
- Minimal histamine release
- Accumulation unlikely even with prolonged infusions

Disadvantages
- Similarly to fentanyl it is a potent respiratory depressant (this may be an advantage in some circumstances) and may cause significant chest wall rigidity

Remifentanil

Synthetic opioid with an analgesic potency of approximately 40 times that of alfentanil.

Advantages
- Very short acting with a rapid onset of action, ideal for using in ventilated patients for dressings changes/physiotherapy, etc., in addition to regular analgesia. For example, a patient may be maintained on a regular background infusion of morphine and then have remifentanil started in addition to this 5–10 minutes before the procedure is starting. This can then be titrated to effect as required with fairly quick results and discontinued after the procedure is completed
- Metabolized by non-specific tissue esterases so metabolism is unaffected by renal function, hepatic function, age, weight, or length of time the patient has been on the drug. It does not accumulate over time and patients wake very predictably
- It is also very potent (analgesic, respiratory suppressant)

Disadvantages
- As it is such a potent respiratory depressant the patient should ideally have a protected airway (endotracheal tube or tracheostomy) and be being supportively ventilated (or be in a position to be if necessary)
- It must not be bloused. It is common practice to bolus analgesic infusions in the critical care setting but due to its profound respiratory depressant effects, remifentanil must not be bloused

Oxycodone

- Synthetic opioid with an oral potency of about one and a half to two times that of oral morphine but a comparable potency when both agents are administered intravenously
- Hepatically metabolized with no active metabolites so a good option in patients with renal failure

Disadvantages
- Currently comparably more expensive than other similar opioids on the market
- Limited experience in its use in the burns population

Methadone

- Useful as an oral alternative for weaning otherwise pain stable patients off other opioids, eg. intravenous morphine. Patients can be switch prior to discharge from intensive care to high dependency beds on burns units
- Has a potency of approximately 5–10 times that of oral morphine (ie. 1 mg of oral methadone is approximately equivalent to 5–10 mg of oral morphine)
- Total daily dose given in two or three divided doses with when necessary doses prescribed at approximately one-sixth of the total daily dose and given at a maximum frequency of every 4 hours during the titration period
- Not to be used for incident pain as onset of action not fast enough

Codeine

- Weak opioid

Advantages
- Cheap

Disadvantages
- Constipating, not particularly potent, it is thought that its analgesic properties predominantly come from the fact that it is metabolized to morphine but up to 10% of white Europeans are slow metabolizers so it is ineffective as an analgesic in this group

Tramadol

Advantages
- May be more effective than other opioids for certain types of pain (for example, bone or neuropathic pain) as it work not only on mu-, kappa- and delta-opioid receptors but also on serotonergic and noradrenergic pathways

Disadvantages
- Described as being a fairly poor analgesic when used as sole therapy (efficacy improved when combined with other agents, eg. paracetamol)
- Lowers seizure threshold
- Nausea and vomiting a common side effect.
- Increases risk of gastrointestinal haemorrhage.
- May cause problematic side effects such as serotonin syndrome if patient is on other drugs affecting serotonin, eg. antidepressants.

Intravenous

Table 47.1 contains guidance on opioid doses used in ventilated patients in the critical care setting; doses would be titrated to effect starting at the lower end of the suggested dosage range.

Many drugs in the critical care setting are prescribed as a standard concentration (see Table 47.10).

Other routes/doses

Table 47.2 provides suggested alternatives to the intravenous infusion for example for incident pain or for when stepping patient down from critical care to a burns unit high dependency.

Fig. 47.1 is an example of a drug monograph used at Whiston Hospital.

Table 47.1 Common opioid dosing regimens used in the intensive care setting

Drug	Bolus	Infusion
Morphine	0.1–0.2 mg/kg	0.05–0.07 mg/kg/h
Fentanyl	1 μg/kg/min for 10 minutes	5–20 μg/kg/h
Alfentanil	15–30 μg/kg	20–120 μg/kg/h
Remifentanil	–	0.25–0.75 μg/kg/min (see example monograph Fig. 47.1)

Table 47.2 Common opioid conversions and doses

Drug	Route	Dose and/or potency
Morphine	Oral	Ratio of 2:1 when converting from intravenous (ie. 10 mg oral approximately equivalent to 5 mg intravenous)
Fentanyl	Topical Buccal/sublingual/ intranasal	25 μg/h patch approximately equivalent to 60–90 mg oral morphine All available as licensed products in the UK, Titrate to effect for incident pain
Alfentanil	Intranasal/buccal	Available as a 1 mg/mL spray, titrate to effect
Oxycodone	Oral	Twice as potent as oral morphine (ie. 10 mg oral morphine approximately equivalent to 5 mg oral oxycodone)
Methadone	Oral	Titrate to effect, see main text
Codeine	Oral	30–60 mg 4–6 hourly, max 240 mg/24 h
Tramadol	Oral	50–100 mg qds prn

REMIFENTANIL – Additional analgesia during dressing changes in
a ventilated burns/plastics patients

PRESENTATION

1 vial contains 5mg REMIFENTANIL as dry powder for reconstitution

INDICATION

**Additional analgesia during dressing changes in a
ventilated burns/plastics patients**

RECONSTITUTION

Dilute 5mg to 50ml with diluent (100micrograms/ml)

DILUENTS

5% glucose intravenous infusion
0.9% sodium chloride intravenous infusion

DOSE

Dose on Idea Body Weight – see notes

**Additional analgesia for ventilated burns/plastics
patients undergoing dressing's changes**

- Initially a rate of at least 0.1micrograms/kg/min should be
  maintained for at least 5minutes prior to the start of the procedure
- Further dose adjustments may be made every 2 to 5 minutes in
  increments of 25%-50%
- Usual maintenance of 0.25micrograms/kg/min
- Usual maximum rate 0.75micrograms/kg/min (can go above this
  at consultants' discretion)
- **Do not give bolus doses.**

INFUSION RATE (mL/hr) using Remifentanil 100micrograms/mL

Idea Body Weight (kg)	Infusion rate (micrograms/kg/min)				
	0.1		0.25		0.75
40	2.4		6		18
50	3	Increase in 25%–50% increments	7.5	Increase in 25%–50% increments	22.5
60	3.6		9		27
70	4.2		10.5		31.5
80	4.8		12		36
90	5.4		13.5		40.5
100	6		15		45

↑	↑	↑
Starting dose	Suggested maintenance	Usual maximum

Fig. 47.1 Example of drug monograph.

Reproduced courtesy of Greg Barton, Specialist Pharmacist Critical Care/Burns, St Helens and
Knowsley Teaching Hospitals NHS Trust.

Non-opioid analgesics

Paracetamol

Advantages
- Cheap, safe (even relatively so in patients with hepatic dysfunction), different action from other analgesics; can be used in combination with other agents to improve both its and their efficacy
- Not just available via the oral route, can also be administered rectally or intravenously

Disadvantages
- Care needed when dosing in patients with a low body weight, in particular with the intravenous preparation. Adults weighing less than 50 kg should have a maximum of 3 g in a 24-hour period

Non-steroidal anti-inflammatory drugs (NSAIDs)

- Avoid were possible in major burn injuries as increase bleeding risk and put added pressure on kidney, liver, and gastrointestinal systems
- Where benefit may outweigh risk, eg. small burn injury with other injuries such as fractured bones, then consider NSAIDs with the best side effect profiles first such as low-dose ibuprofen (400 mg tds) or naproxen 250–500 mg bd

Drug for neuropathic pain

- Partial thickness burns and graft donor sites in some patients cause them the most discomfort. Exposed and damaged nerves may lead to longstanding pain that is relatively resistant to standard therapies such as opioids or paracetamol. Options include the following.

Gabapentin/pregabalin
- Binds at voltage-dependent Ca^{2+} channels to increase the amount of GABA in the synapse
- Analgesic but also improves sleep in patients with neuropathic pain
- Works synergistically to increases the effects of morphine
- Pregabalin is a pro-drug of gabapentin
- Side effects common at higher doses and may limit usefulness/compliance

Amitriptyline
- Tricyclic antidepressants have long been used to treat neuropathic pain
- Unlicensed

Lidocaine patches
- Should only be used on healed areas but may be beneficial in residual neuropathic pain and add in allowing patients to tolerate physiotherapy and mobilization

Ketamine

- Ketamine is primarily a dissociative anaesthetic but can also be used for the management of chronic pain. It main mode of action is as a non-competitive antagonist of NMDA receptors but some its analgesic properties may be due to modulation of opioid receptors
- It can be used as a sedative in the intensive care setting or as a adjunct to other analgesics such as opioid infusions during painful procedures like dressings changes
- In the more chronic phase of pain it can be used with specialist guidance intravenously in a PCA or as an oral regimen

Dosing guidance

Table 47.3 provides guidance on dosing regimens for non-opioid analgesics.

Table 47.3 Dosing regimens for non-opioid analgesics

Drug	Dose
Paracetamol	500 mg to 1 g 4–6 hourly regular or when required, max 4 g/24 h (3 g/24 h if body weight <50 kg); oral/intravenous
NSAIDs	
Ibuprofen	200–400 mg 6–8 hourly regular or when required; oral
Naproxen	250–500 mg bd regular or when required; oral
Drugs for neuropathic pain	
Gabapentin	300 mg on day 1, 300 mg on day 2, then 300 mg tds thereafter. Can be further titrated, maximum licensed dose 3.6 g/24 h but higher doses have been used under specialist advice.
Pregabalin	Initially 150 mg in 2–3 divided doses; maximum dose 600 mg/24 h
Amitriptyline	Initially 10 mg nocte, maximum 75 mg daily
Lidocaine patch	1–3 patches applied to the affected areas for 12 hours each day
Ketamine	Seek specialist advice locally
	For example, may be administered as patient controlled analgesia (PCA) as 1-mg boluses with a 5-minute lock out or if the oral route is available start at 10 mg tds

Sedatives

- The following drugs should only be used in the patients with a protected airway, ie. intubated patients in a critical care setting
- Sedative doses should generally be titrated to effect against regular (daily) sedation breaks where appropriate or a sedation scoring system such as the Ramsey scale or the Richmond Agitation Sedation Scale (RASS)

Propofol

- Used commonly as a first line sedative on critical care throughout the UK
- Intravenous anaesthetic. Mode of action unclear, potentiates glycine and GABA

Advantages

- Short duration of action (starts and stops quickly); half-life approximately 10–70 minutes with less accumulation than other sedative drugs
- Good for assessing the patient, eg. head injury
- Anti-tussive/reduces bronchospasm

Disadvantages

- Only licensed for 3 days
- More expensive than some other agents
- Tolerance may develop
- High lipid load (1% preparation contains 1 kcal/mL; monitor triglycerides)
- Contraindicated in children
- Causes hypotension: reduces blood pressure by 15–25% without a compensatory rise in cardiac output
- No analgesic effects
- Peanut allergy
- Propofol infusion syndrome

Benzodiazepines

- Benzodiazepine, acts at benzodiazepine receptors linked to GABA receptors
- Midazolam is commonly the drug of choice in UK critical care units

Advantages

- Short acting: half life approximately 2 hours
- Respiratory depression
- Anterograde amnesia
- Cheaper?

Disadvantages

- Respiratory depression.
- Anterograde amnesia.
- Accumulation (especially in renal impairment)
- Hypotension?
- No analgesic effects

Selective α_2 receptor agonists, eg. clonidine or dexmedetomidine

- Have their analgesic effects predominantly centrally, eg. at the dorsal horn of the spinal cord
- Act as analgesic and sedation/analgesic-sparing effects
- May cause less sedation-induced delirium than other agents such as benzodiazepines
- Dexmedetomidine is newly licensed in the UK and as yet there is very limited experience with its use in the burns population; it is more potent sedative than clonidine but it has less analgesic properties (and less effects on blood pressure)

Sedatives and their suggested dosage ranges

Table 47.4 highlights the standard dose ranges used for intubated patient in the intensive care setting. These drugs are usually titrated to a sedation score (see example in Table 47.5).

Monitoring sedation

Table 47.5 describes a sedation score used on Whiston hospital intensive care unit to monitor the patient's responsiveness while sedated. The target generally is 1 (aware but calm) but there are instances in the management of the burns patient, eg. dressings changes or passive limb movements during physiotherapy where a lower score may be more appropriate to reduce patient distress.

Table 47.4 Standard dosage ranges for common sedatives in intensive care

Drug	Dose
Propofol	1–4 mg/kg/h; maximum dose 4 mg/kg/h
Midazolam	10–50 µg/kg/min
Clonidine	Initially start at 1 µg/kg/h
	Increase by increments of 0.5 mL/h every 3 hours if BP stable
	max dose 4 µg/kg/h
	When discontinuing, wean gradually over a number of hours (eg. reduce by 50% every 2 hours). If hypertension occurs reduce rate more slowly
Dexmedetomidine	Initially 0.7 µg/kg/h; usual range 0.2–1.4 µg/kg/h. Make adjustments in rate hourly until required sedation level is achieved

Table 47.5 Whiston hospitals sedation score

3	Agitated and restless
2	Awake and uncomfortable
1	Aware but calm
0	Roused by voice, calm
−1	Roused by movement
−2	Roused by pain
−3	Unrousable
A	Natural sleep
P	Paralysed

Fluids

- Fluids play an important role starting immediately post-burn injury right through the patients hospital stay
- Initial fluid resuscitation is achieved with following a set protocol such as Parkland's (using Hartmann's/Ringers lactate solution) or Muir Barkley (using albumin)
- To avoid overhydration the resuscitation fluid rate can be modified targeting a specific urine output. For example 0.5–1 mL/pre-burn kg/h
- It may be necessary to prescribe a regimen of background fluid on top of the resuscitation fluid, eg. an extra 2–3 L of Hartmanns/Ringers lactate or 4% glucose/0.18% sodium chloride
- Additional fluid boluses may be required to maintain blood pressure, it is as yet unclear as to whether these fluid boluses should be crystalloid (Hartmanns/Ringers lactate) or colloid (such as gelatine or starch). If fluid boluses alone are not enough or appropriate consider starting a vasopressor such as noradrenaline (noradrenaline (norepinephrine))
- It may be appropriate to use hypertonic albumin solutions to replace low serum albumin levels targeting for example a level of 20 g/L or greater

Vasopressors

- Before starting vasopressors make sure the patient is adequately filled with fluid (see Parklands Formulary, Muir Barkley Formulary).

Noradrenaline

- Acts predominantly on α_1 receptors (agonist) although has some β_1 action
- An extremely potent vasopressor
- Cardiovascular effects
- ↑ BP (and SVR) via arterial and venous vasoconstriction
- Cardiac output may ↑ or ↓ depending on clinical circumstances
- Cautions. Acts by increasing afterload; not appropriate for use in patients with cardiogenic shock (blood supply to kidneys and peripheries may be decreased)

Vasopressin

- Synthetic copy of a naturally occurring peptide hormone
- Vasopressin agonist
- Vasoconstrictor (via AVP receptor 1A).
- Used as an adjunct to therapy (usually combined with NA) (Table 47.6)

Table 47.6 Standard starting doses for vasopressors

Drug	Dose
Noradrenaline	Start infusion at 0.05 µg/kg/min but can be titrated quickly to achieve target blood pressure
Vasopressin	Start at 0.03 units/minute, reduce cautiously once target blood pressure has been achieved

Stress ulcer prophylaxis

Stress ulceration has historically been a common complication in the major burns patient but improved nursing care, early enteral feeding and changes in practice such as 30° head of the bed elevation have helped greatly reduce its incidence. Drugs interventions are however still regularly prescribed.

Sucralfate

- A complex of aluminium hydroxide and sulphated sucrose
- May act to prevent stress ulceration by protecting the stomach mucosa from acid pepsin attack
- There have been reports of bezoar formation lead to some text advising caution in its use in the critically ill especially those being enteraly feed or with delayed gastric emptying
- May cause less nosocomial pneumonias and *Clostridium difficile* diarrhoeas than H_2 antagonist and proton pump inhibitors but evidence of this is debatable
- Likely to cause constipation and may impede absorption of some drugs, eg. digoxin if given at the same time
- Falling out of favour

H_2 antagonists

- Eg. Ranitidine
- Inhibit secretion of gastric acid by antagonism of histamine h_2 receptors
- Given intravenously or oral/enterally

Proton pump inhibitors

- Eg. omeprazole (IV or ng/oral), pantoprazole (IV or ng/oral) or lansoprazole (ng/oral)
- Inhibit gastric acid secretion by inhibiting H^+K^+-atpase
- May carry an increased risk of ventilator associated pneumonia and *Clostridium difficile* infection compared to the other agents but evidence in inconclusive
- Can be given enterally or intravenously
- Lansoprazole orodispersible tablets can potentially block fine bore feeding tubes so other preparations may be more suitable to be administered by the nasogastric route

Common doses

Table 47.7 Common drugs and dosages prescribed for stress ulcer prophylaxis

Drug	Dose
Sucralfate	Oral/enteral 1 g 4–6 hourly
Ranitidine	IV 50 mg tds Oral/enteral 150 mg bd
Proton pump inhibitors	Oral/enteral lansoprazole 30 mg od IV pantoprazole/omeprazole 40 mg od

Vitamins, amino acids, and trace elements

Replacement of deficiencies of certain vitamins and trace elements may be beneficial in aiding wound healing. The following all have some evidence to suggest supplementation may be of benefit to the patient but exact targets and doses are as yet unclear (Table 47.8).

- Ascorbic acid
- Zinc
- Selenium
- Glutamine
- Copper

Table 47.8 Suggested dosing regimens (enterally)

Dose	Example dosing regimen
Ascorbic acid	100 mg tds up to 1 g daily
Zinc sulfate	125 mg tds
Copper	2 mg daily
Selenium	200 μg daily
Glutamine	0.3 g/kg/day *intravenously* for 5–10 days

Antibiotics

- Generic or prophylactic antibiotics are generally not indicated
- Body temperature often rises as high as 40°C in the first day or two in major burns, and may persist for a week or so. This is not necessarily indicative of a secondary infection
- Antibiotic therapy should be guided by a combination of clinically suspected infection site, serum inflammatory markers (eg. white cell count, C-reactive protein) and ideally cultures and sensitivities if available
- Although the burn area is a highly susceptible to infection, regular dressings, topical antiseptics, baths, and good nursing care reduce the likelihood of this
- The respiratory system is a likely source, especially in the ventilated patient who may have an undiagnosed/unmeasurable airway burn; even without an airway injury intubated patients are also at risk of ventilator-associated pneumonia. Systemic digestive tract decontamination (SDD) should be considered, this consists of a combination of oral +/− intravenous antibiotics used prophylactically to eradicate potentially harmful normal gut floral. It is generally an infection control strategy applied to the whole Intensive Care Unit but may still work where burns patients are nursed in isolation/cubicles. See Box 47.1 for an example regimen
- Antibiotic dosing is very important in the major burn injury as the pharmacokinetics can be very different from the standard patient
- During the initial acute phase diffuse increases in capillary permeability throughout the body lead to the loss of protein rich fluid, this in turn can lead to a drop in cardiac output causing end organ hypoperfusion. For example reduction in blood flow to the kidneys will transpire as a reduction in glomerular filtration rate and potentially a reduction in removal of renally cleared drugs
- After approximately 48 hours the patient enters a catabolic phase assuming they have been adequately volume resuscitated and so have an increased cardiac output with a corresponding increase in renal and hepatic blood flows
- During both of these phases antibiotic pharmacokinetics will be altered and different dosing strategies should be considered such as doses above the normal licensed dose or extended infusion administration practices (eg. each dose of piperacillin/tazobactam or meropenem infused over 3 or 4 hours or vancomycin given as a continuous infusion). Where possible therapeutic drug monitoring should be used for all antibiotics to target dosing/administration effectively.

Box 47.1 Example of systemic digestive tract decontamination (SDD) protocol

- SDD paste/gel (topically to the gums and lips of intubated and additionally the tracheostomy site in tracheotomized patients)
- Colistimethate sodium 50 mg/mL; 2 mL qds ng
- Amphotericin 100 mg/mL; 5 mL qds ng
- Tobramycin 27 mg/mL; 2 mL qds ng
- +/− intravenous broad-spectrum antibiotic such as a cephalosporin

Fluid-sparing drugs

Some drugs, eg. ascorbic acid, if started soon after burn injury, are thought to reduce the amount of fluid required in the resuscitation stage after a burn injury. However, their incorporation into standard practice has so far been limited by lack of evidence and practical aspects such as availability of a suitable intravenous preparation

Muscle-sparing drugs (anticatabolic measures)

Used in the phase of increased metabolic rate and hyperdynamic circulation post burn injury to prevent accelerated muscle wasting that may delay mobilization and therefore impede recovery and even increasing mortality.

Propranolol

- A beta-blocker that acts by competitive antagonism of both beta 1 and beta 2 adrenoceptors. Reduces heart rate (tachycardia), thermogenesis and resting energy expenditure. It also increases lean body mass and reduces skeletal muscle wasting
- In practice start at a low dose for example 10 mg bd and then titrate rapidly to attain a heart rate of between 60 and 100 beats per minute, usual dosage range 10–40 mg bd–tds
- Therapy with propranolol is often interrupted or contraindicated as hypotension in septic or otherwise haemodynamically unstable patients results in the use of vasopressors (such as noradrenaline), which limits it role

Anabolic steroids

- Used primarily to prevent muscle wasting

Oxandrolone

- 1/20th the potency of testosterone, indicated for use in both male and female patients
- Key trial suggests 10 mg bd enterally starting on day 5 after burn injury and continuing until hospital discharge
- There is no specific target or monitoring of effectiveness, can be used while patient is on vasopressors. Liver function tests (specifically transaminases) should be monitored and oxandralone discontinued if significant anomaly occurs
- No preparation is readily available in the UK; a licensed preparation is available in the USA

Nandrolone

- Used as an alternative to oxandrolone because it is more easily available in the UK
- Insulin, metformin, and other agents that reduce post-burn hyperglycaemia may be of benefit
- Consider also non-pharmacological interventions such as adequate enteral feeding (at 35 kcal/kg/day during the catabolic phase with a high protein feed such as Jevity® Plus HP) and a high ambient room temperature (28–30°C)

Itch

- During healing of partial thickness burns or donor sites itch can be a problematic complication
- A combination of antihistamines and topical cooling agents may be most effective
- Calamine lotion is alcohol based and so can cause drying of the skin and irritation in itself so is best avoided
- In general sedating antihistamines are more effective than non-sedating but may not be practical during the day therefore a regimen of non-sedating antihistamines such a fexofenadine during the day supplemented with a sedating agent such as hydroxyzine at night may work
- 1% menthol in aqueous cream applied liberally when required is a suitable and effective topical agent (Tables 47.9 and 47.10)

Table 47.9 Examples of antihistamine oral dosing regimens

Drug	Dose
Chlorphenamine	4 mg 4 hourly, maximum 24 mg/24 h
Hydroxyzine	10 mg bd and 25 mg nocte
Fexofenadine and hydroxyzine combination	120 mg fexofenadine in a morning and 25 mg hydroxyzine nocte

Suggested drug concentrations

Table 47.10 Suggested standard drug concentrations in the UK as supported by the United Kingdom Clinical Pharmacy Association (UKCPA) and Intensive Care Society (ICS)

Medication	Infusion composition	Concentration
Morphine	50 mg in 50 mL	1 mg/mL
	100 mg in 50 mL	2 mg/mL
Fentanyl	2.5 mg in 50 mL	50 µg/mL
Alfentanil	25 mg in 50 mL	500 µg/mL
Remifentanil	2 mg in 40 mL	50 µg/mL
	5 mg in 50 mL	100 µg/mL
Midazolam	50 mg in 50 mL	1 mg/mL
	100 mg in 50 mL	2 mg/mL
Clonidine	750µg in 50 mL	15 µg/mL
Dexmedetomidine	200µg in 50 mL	4 µg/mL
	400µg in 50 mL	8 µg/mL
Adrenaline	4 mg in 50 mL	80 µg/mL
	8 mg in 50 mL	160 µg/mL
	16 mg in 50 mL	320 µg/mL
	8 mg in 100 mL	80 µg/mL
	16 mg in 100 mL	160 µg/mL
	32 mg in 100 mL	320 µg/mL
Noradrenaline	4 mg in 50 mL	80 µg/mL
	8 mg in 50 mL	160 µg/mL
	16 mg in 50 mL	320 µg/mL
	8 mg in 100 mL	80 µg/mL
	16 mg in 100 mL	160 µg/mL
	32 mg in 100 mL	320 µg/mL
Dobutamine	250 mg in 50 mL	5 mg/mL
	500 mg in 100 mL	5 mg/mL
Dopamine	200 mg in 50 mL	4 mg/mL
	400 mg in 50 mL	8 mg/mL
Vasopressin (Argipressin)	20 units in 50 mL	0.4 units/mL
Amiodarone (load)	300 mg in 50 mL	6 mg/mL
	300 mg in 100 mL	3 mg/mL

(Continued)

Table 47.10 (*Contd.*)

Medication	Infusion composition	Concentration
Amiodarone (continuation …)	300 mg in 50 mL	6 mg/mL
	600 mg in 50 mL	12 mg/mL
	900 mg in 50 mL	18 mg/mL
	300 mg in 500 mL	0.6 mg/mL
	600 mg in 500 mL	1.2 mg/mL
	900 mg in 500 mL	1.8 mg/mL
Heparin	20,000 units in 20 mL	1,000 units/mL
	25,000 units in 25 mL	1,000 units/mL
Magnesium sulfate	20 mmol in 50 mL	0.4 mmol/mL
	20 mmol in 100 mL	0.2 mmol/mL
	20 mmol in 250 mL	0.08 mmol/mL
Phosphate	20 mmol in 50 mL	0.4 mmol/mL
	40 mmol in 100 mL	0.4 mmol/mL
	50 mmol in 500 mL	0.1 mmol/mL
Insulin	50 units in 50 mL	1 unit/mL
Epoprostenol	The formulation of Flolan® has changed. Different formulations in circulation. Consult package insert.	

Reproduced with the kind permission of the Intensive Care Society and the Faculty of Intensive Care Medicine.

Further reading

Ali A, Herndon DN, Mamachen A, et al. Propranolol attenuates hemorrhage and accelerates wound healing in severely burned adults. Critical Care 2015;19:217.

Bull JP, Squire JR. A study of mortality in a burns unit. Annals of Surgery, 1949;160–73.

Demling RH, DeSanti L. The rate of restoration of body weight after burn injury, using the anabolic agent oxandrolone, is not age dependent. Burns 2001;27:46–51.

Demling RH, Orgill DP. The anticatabolic and wound healing effects of the testosterone analog oxandrolone after severe burn injury. Journal of Critical Care 2000;15:12–17.

Demling RH, DeSanti L. Oxandrolone induced lean mass gain during recovery from severe burns is maintained after discontinuation of the anabolic steroid. Burns 2003;29:793–7.

Jeschke MG, Herndon DN. Burns in children: standard and new treatments. Lancet 2014;383:1168–78.

Lundy JB, Chung KK, Pamplin JC, et al. Update on severe burn management for the intensivist. Journal of Intensive Care Medicine 2016;31:499–510.

Navickis RJ, Greenhalgh DG, Wilkes MM. Albumin in burn shock resuscitation: a meta-analysis of controlled clinical studies. Journal of Burn Care & Research 2016;37:e268–78.

Nordlund MJ, Pham TN, Gibran NS. Micronutrients after burn injury: a review. Journal of Burn Care & Research 2014;35:121–33.

Richardson P, Mustard L. The management of pain in the burns unit. Burns 2009;35:921–36.

Rousseau A-F, Losser M-R, Ichai C, Berger MM. ESPEN endorsed recommendations: nutritional therapy in major burns. Clinical Nutrition 2013;32, 497–502.

Rowan MP, Cancio LC, Elster EA, et al. Burn wound healing and treatment: review and advancements. Critical Care 2015;19:243.

Sánchez-Sánchez M, Garcia-de-Lorenzo A, Herrero E, et al. Evaluation of a protocol for resuscitation in burn patients. Critical Care 2014;18:430.

Sánchez M, García-de-Lorenzo A, Herrero E, et al. A protocol for resuscitation of severe burn patients guided by transpulmonary thermodilution and lactate levels: a 3-year prospective cohort study. Critical Care 2013;17:R176.

Sen S, Greenhalgh D, Palmieri T. Review of burn injury research for the year 2009. Journal of Burn Care & Research 2010;31:836–48.

Sen S, Palmieri T, Greenhalgh D. Review of burn research for the year 2013. Journal of Burn Care & Research 2014;35:362–8.

Summer GJ, Puntillo KA, Miaskowski C, et al. Burn injury pain: the continuing challenge. Journal of Pain 2007;8:533–48.

Tran NK, Godwin ZR, Bockhold JC, et al. Clinical impact of sample interference on intensive insulin therapy in severely burned patients: a pilot study. Journal of Burn Care & Research 2009;35:72–9.

Walker PF, Buehner MF, Wood LA, et al. Diagnosis and management of inhalation injury: an updated review. Critical Care 2015;19:351.

Weinbren MJ. Pharmacokinetics of antibiotics in burn patients. Journal of Antimicrobial Chemotherapy 1999;44:319–27.

Transfer proforma

Transfer proforma: part 1

Patient name	DoB and age	Weight (kg)

Date and time of burn	History of injury
Date and time arrived to primary unit	
Referring unit: Referrer name: Grade: Direct line: Fax number:	Other injuries
Details of first aid	Allergies tetanus status

Past medical history (including medications, smoking, alcohol, occupation, psychiatric history)

BURN TBSA% CHART

Ignore simple erythema

Draw what is described

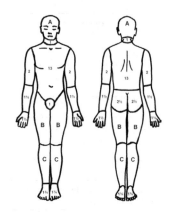

Estimated Burn TBSA
=   %

Area	Age 0	1	5	10	15	Adult
A= ½ of head	9½	8½	6½	5½	4½	3½
B= ½ of one thigh	2¾	3¼	4	4½	4½	4¾
C= ½ of one lower leg	2½	2½	2¾	3	3¼	3½

Body region	Partial thickness (%)	Full thickness (%)
Head		
Neck		
Anterior trunk		
Posterior trunk		
Right arm		
Left arm		
Buttocks		
Genitalia		
Right leg		
Left leg		
Total Burn		

Wound management advice
Language: Is an interpreter needed: Yes/No
Next of kin (name, relationship, and contact details)
Referral accepted/declined for transfer (N.B. check if ITU bed available, if required)
If accepted for transfer and TBSA >15%, tick when transfer proforma – part 2 faxed to referring unit for completion ☐
Form completed by (sign and print) Designation Contact details

© Susie Zhi-Jie Yao with kind permission

Transfer proforma: part 2

Patient name	DoB and age	Weight (kg)

Airway/breathing

SpO^2 %   RR   /min   FiO^2 %

Inhalation injury   Yes/No

Seen by anesthetist   Yes/No
Name and grade

Intubation   Yes/No

Laryngoscopy grade   I II III IV

Size ETT   cuffed/uncuffed

Pre-intubation GCS

C-spine immobilized   Yes/No

If no, name and grade who cleared C-spine

Circulation

HR   /min   BP /   Cap refill   sec

Site and size of IV cannulae

1

2

Fluid resus commenced   Yes/No

Core temperature   °C

Urinary catheter   Yes/No

ATLS primary survey done   Yes/No
ATLS secondary survey done   Yes/No
Performed by

Fluid resuscitation (for adults >15% TBSA burn, children >10% TBSA burn only)

For the first 24 hours (Parkland's formula):

2–4 mL Hartmann's solution per % burn per kg, half over first 8 hours, from time of injury not presentation:

Higher fluid is used for severe inhalational injury, lower for significant pathology such as heart failure. A tailored response to urine output is important. Therefore, a catch-up bolus may be required liaison with accepting unit is critical (**check calculations with accepting unit**).

We expect the patient to be transferred to the burn unit within 8 hours.

Paediatric fluid resuscitation: in addition to these fluids, paediatric shock burn patients also require maintenance fluids using a dextrose/saline solution such as 5% dextrose & 0.45% sodium chloride at a volume of:
100 mL/kg for the first 10 kg plus ...
50 mL/kg for the second 10 kg plus ...
20 mL/kg for each additional kg
The total given over 24 hours

Fluid balance chart – please complete with ACTUAL volumes for each hour. Aim for urine output of 0.5–1 mL/kg/h

Time from burn injury	Hartmann's (mL)	Other IV fluids (mL)	Oral fluids (mL)	Urine output (mL)
Hour 1				
Hour 2				
Hour 3				
Hour 4				
Hour 5				
Hour 6				
Hour 7				
Hour 8				

Time	Medication Given	Dose	Route

Other tests/imaging with results

TESTS		ABG	
Hb		pH	
WBC		pO_2	
Plts		pCO_2	
Na^+		HCOs	
K^+		BE	

Urea		Lactate	
Creatinine		CoHB%	
Albumin			
Glucose		Create kinase	
ECG			

Pre-transfer check list (tick or n/a)	
Airway safe/secure	
Tubes/lines secure	
Catheter taped	
Warming in place	
Analgesia adequate	
Fluid continued in transit	
Appropriate staff for transfer	
Jewellery etc. removed	
Notes/imaging	
Blood results	
Relative aware	
Time of departure	

Form completed by (sign and print)

Designation
Contact details

Burn care referral criteria

United Kingdom national network for burn care referral criteria

All injuries deemed complex should be discussed with the regional burns unit, and in most cases referred for assessment or management. Irrespective of these criteria, if a referring team is unsure about any burns injury, they should discuss the case with the burns specialist team.[1]

Complex burn

A burn injury is more likely to be complex if associated with the following criteria:

Age	<5 years or >60 years
Burn size	<16 years, TBSA >5% or >16 years, TBSA >10%
Burn location	Face, hands, perineum, feet, any flexure (esp. neck/axilla)
Circumferential injury	Any circumferential burns of limbs/torso/neck (risk of compartment syndrome)
Inhalation injury	Any significant such injury with/without cutaneous burn (excluding pure carbon monoxide poisoning)
Mechanism of injury	Chemical injury (>5% TBSA) Hydrofluoric acid injury (>1% TBSA) Exposure to ionizing radiation injury High pressure steam injury High tension electrical injury Suspicion of non-accidental burn injury (adult/paediatric)
Pre-existing conditions eg.	Cardiac limitation +/– MI <5 years Respirator limitation of exercise Diabetes Pregnancy Immune suppression Hepatic impairment, cirrhosis
Associated injuries	Crush injuries Fractures Head injury Penetrating injuries
Vesiculobullous disorders eg.	Any of these diseases affecting >5% TBSA Epidermolysis bullosa Staphylococcal scalded skin syndrome (Ritter's) Stevens–Johnson syndrome Toxic epidermal necrolysis (Lyell's)

It is at the discretion of the accepting doctor whether the patient needs urgent transfer to the ward or can be more appropriately reviewed at a later date/time

Data sourced from NHS Specialised Services National Network for Burn Care (NNBC), National Burn Care Referral Guidance, Version 1, Approved February 2012, Copyright © National Network for Burn Care (NNBC), available from https://www.britishburnassociation.org/national-burn-care-referral-guidance/

References

1. NHS Specialised Services National Network for Burn Care (NNBC), National Burn Care Referral Guidance, Version 1, Approved February 2012, https://www.britishburnassociation. org/wp-content/uploads/2018/02/National-Burn-Care-Referral-Guidance-2012.pdf (accessed 2 October 2018).

Admission proforma

Admission proforma

Referring unit	Patient name	Age
Date at clerking		Weight (kg)
Time at clerking	DOB	Time patient arrived on Burns Unit
Location at clerking	Hospital number	

Mechanism of injury

Flame	☐	Cold	☐
Flash	☐	Electrical	☐
Scald	☐	Chemical	☐
Contact	☐	Radiation	☐
Friction	☐	Other (specify):	

Inhalation injury: Yes/No   Intubated: Yes/No

Date and time of burn

History of injury (resuscitation if >15% TBSA or >10% in child)

Alcohol involved: Yes / No   Drugs involved: Yes / No
Fire-brigade involved: Yes / No   Enclosed space: Yes / No
Associated injuries:

Details of first aid (type and timing):

Medications

Allergies   Tetanus covered: Yes/No
                         Tetanus immunoglobulin given: Yes/No

Past medical History (including psychiatric history)

Social history

Smoking: Alcohol: Recreational drugs:
  cig/day   units/wk

Occupation: Home situation: Hand dominance:
                                     Right/Left

Mobility:

Examination

Airway/breathing

SpO_2 %   RR   /min FiO_2 %

Inhalation injury   Yes/No

Seen by anaesthetist   Yes/No
Name and grade

Intubation   Yes/No

C-spine immobilized   Yes/No

If No, name agrade who cleared C-spine

Circulation

HR   /min   BP /   Cap refill   sec

Site and size of peripheral and central lines

1

2

Fluid resuscitation commenced   Yes/No

Urinary catheterisation   Yes/No

Blood glucose   mmol/L

Core temperature   °C

ATLS primary survey done   Yes/No
ATLS secondary survey done   Yes/No
Performed by

BURN TBSA% CHART

Ignore simple erythema

Draw what is described

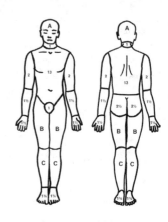

| Estimated Burn TBSA |
| = % |

Area	Age 0	1	5	10	15	Adult
A= ½ of head	9½	8½	6½	5½	4½	3½
B= ½ of one thigh	2¾	3¼	4	4½	4½	4¾
C= ½ of one lower leg	2½	2½	2¾	3	3¼	3½

Body region	Partial thickness (%)	Full thickness (%)
Head		
Neck		
Anterior trunk		
Posterior trunk		
Right arm		
Left arm		
Buttocks		
Genitalia		
Right leg		
Left leg		
Total Burn		

Abdominal examination

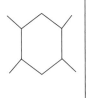

Other injury specific examination findings (e.g. eyes, ears)

Blood results

Electrocardiogram

Chest radiograph

Other investigations

Plan

Use separate sheet if required for resuscitation fluids
(TBSA >15% or >10% in child)

Standard burns drug regimen:

Mechanical thromboprophylaxis: Yes/No
Pharmacological thromboprophylaxis: Yes/No
Gastric Protection: Yes/No
Analgesia: Yes/No

Multivitamins and other supplements: Yes/No

Form completed by (sign and print name)

Designation and
Contact details

Burn links

Burn Associations

British Burn Association
35–43 Lincoln's Inn Fields, London, WC2A 3PE, UK
T: 020 7869 6923
F: 020 7869 6929
E: info@britishburnassociation.org
www.britishburnassociation.org

American Burn Association
ABA Central office, 311 S. Wacker Drive, Suite 4150, Chicago, IL
60606, USA
T: (312) 642-9260
F: (312) 642-9130
E: info@ameriburn.org
http://www.ameriburn.org

Australian and New Zealand Burn Association
PO Box 550, Albany Creek, QLD 4035, Australia
T: +61 7 3325 1030
F: +61 7 3325 1042
E: info@anzba.org.au
www.anzba.org.au

Pan African Burn Society
http://www.pabs.co.za

European Burns Association
P.O. Box 1015, 1940 EA Beverwijk, The Netherlands
E: info@euroburn.org
F: +31(0)251 224408
www.euroburn.org

International Society for Burn Injuries
Elisabeth Greenfield, RN, MSN, 2172 US Highway 181 South,
Floresville, TX 781114, USA
E: lizals@tgti.net
www.worldburn.org

Interburns
Tom Potokar, Interburns, Welsh Centre for Burns and Plastic Surgery,
Swansea, SA6 6NL, Wales, UK
E: office@interburns.org
www.interburns.org

Research Bodies

The Healing Foundation
The Royal College of Surgeons of England, 35 - 43 Lincoln's Inn Fields, London, WC2A 3PE, UK
T: 020 7869 6920
F: 020 7869 6929
E: info@thehealingfoundation.org
www.thehealingfoundation.org

The Wound Healing Society
341 N. Maitland Ave., Suite 130, Maitland, Florida 32751, USA
T: +1 407-647-8839
E: info@woundheal.org
www.woundheal.org

The Surgical Materials Testing Laboratory (SMTL)
Princess of Wales Hospital Coity Road, Bridgend, South Wales, CF31 1RQ, UK
T: 01656 752820
F: 01656 752830
E: info@smtl.co.uk
www.smtl.co.uk

Tissue Viability Society
c/o Professor Jane Nixon, Clinical Trials Research Unit (CTRU)
University of Leeds, Leeds, LS2 9JT, UK
www.tvs.org.uk

Trauma Audit and Research Network (TARN)
Manchester Medical Academic Health Sciences Centre
University of Manchester, 3rd Floor, The Mayo Building
Salford Royal NHS Foundation Trust, Stott Lane, Salford
M6 8HD, UK
T: 0161 206 4397
F: 0161 206 4345
E: support@tarn.ac.uk
www.tarn.ac.uk

European Tissue Repair Society
Rue Cingria 7, Geneva, CH-1205, Switzerland
T: +41 22 321 48 90
F: +41 22 321 48 92
www.etrs.org

European Wound Management Association
EWMA Secretariat, Nordre Fasanvej 113, 2. DK-2000 Frederiksberg, Denmark
T: +45 70 20 03 05
F: +45 70 20 03 15
E: ewma@ewma.org
www.ewma.org

Scar Club
http://www.scar-club.com/

UK Charities

The Katie Piper Foundation
Katie Piper Foundation, Building 3, Chiswick Park, 566 Chiswick High Road,
Chiswick, London W4 5YA, United Kingdom.
http://www.katiepiperfoundation.org.uk/

Children's Burns Trust
38 Buckingham Place Road, London. SW1W 0RE
T: 020 7233 8333
F: 020 7233 8200
E: info@cbtrust.org.uk
www.cbtrust.org.uk

Dan's Fund for Burns
PO Box 54394, London,W2 7HJ,UK
T: 020 7262 4039
F: 020 7262 8546
E: info@dansfundforburns.org
www.dansfundforburns.org

Children's Burns Foundation
4th Floor, MacLaren House, Lancastrian Office Centre, Talbot Road,
Manchester, M32 0FP, UK
T: 0161 359 3474
F: 0161 872 2777
E: enq@cbf-uk.org
www.cbf-uk.org

The Burned Children's Club
28 Malyons Place, Basildon, Essex, SS13 1PS, UK
T: 0268-527-796
M: 07876-636-415
E: burncamp@tiscali.co.uk
www.burnedchildrensclub.org.uk

British Association of Skin Camouflage
PO Box 3671, Chester, Cheshire, CH1 9QH, UK
T: 01254 703 107
http://www.skin-camouflage.net

Changing Faces
The Squire Centre, 33-37 University Street, London, WC1E 6JN, UK.
T: 0845 4500 275 or 0207 391 9270.
F: 0845 4500 276
E: info@changingfaces.org.uk
www.changingfaces.org.uk

Burn Support Group Database
http://www.burnsupportgroupsdatabase.com

Research Journals

Scars, Burns & Healing (SAGE)
https://uk.sagepub.com/en-gb/eur/scars-burns-healing/journal202486

Burns (Elsevier)
http://www.journals.elsevier.com/burns/

Journal of Burn Care and Research (LWW)
http://journals.lww.com/burncareresearch/pages/default.aspx

Index

Figures, tables and boxes are indicated by an italic *f*, *t* or *b* following the page number.